Baby's First Year

Paulien Bom and Machteld Huber

Baby's First Year

Growth and Development from 0 to 12 Months

Written in cooperation with Guus van der Bie,
Toke Bezuijen, Anneke Maissan and Paul Wormer

Floris Books

Translated by Tony Langham and Plym Peters

Originally published in Dutch under the title
Groeiwijzer van nul tot één jaar by Christofoor in 1994
Sixth Dutch edition published in 2006

First published in English in 2008 by Floris Books, Edinburgh.

British Library CIP Data available

ISBN 978-086315-633-5

Printed in Great Britain by
Athenaeum Press, Gateshead

Contents

Foreword

As a practising anthroposophical doctor, it was with pleasure that I was asked to check the translation of this book. Reading it brought back many memories of looking after a newborn baby: the warmth of holding a little bundle; the miracle of the first smile; the endless new achievements, and the overwhelming love for a child.

What I also recalled was the trauma of a difficult birth, severe exhaustion, anxiety about being a good enough parent, and the worry of creating a perfect environment for my baby. I need not have worried; children do grow up and are, with some careful nurturing, quite robust.

Parents and carers will find a wealth of information in this small book, about how to nurture babies in a natural, wholesome way. The information is the result of years of practical experience gleaned from many health professionals, who have worked in specialist baby clinics in Holland. The advice given in this book is also practised in University clinics in Germany.

Take the advice in this book as a collection of good ideas, some of which you will manage to make your own, others not. Many new parents experience a range of conflicting emotions: maybe the birth was not the idyllic home water-birth you had hoped for; maybe you are quite stressed and tired, or maybe you can't find organic baby food.

At the end of day, a parent's love and consistency are the most important things a child needs.

Marga Hogenboom, 2008

About the authors

Guus van der Bie is a doctor at the Centre for Anthroposophical Health Care, Zeist, Holland, where he has a clinic. He is also active in anthroposophical medical research and training.

Paulien Bom-Bos worked for years as a nurse at an anthroposophical health centre in Amsterdam and at the clinic of the Centre for Anthroposophical Health Care, Zeist. She now works as publicist.

Machteld Huber is a doctor, and was the Director of the Dunamis Institute for ten years, providing general information on health as well as organic food, which resulted in the idea for this book. Presently, she is researching organic food quality and health.

Toke Bezuijen works as a nurse practitioner at the Centre for Anthroposophical Health Care, Zoetermeer. In addition, she gives courses on the care and upbringing of infants and toddlers, and organizes antenatal courses. She also works as a therapist, providing physical and palliative treatments in her own practice, as well as at the Centre for Anthroposophical Health Care in Leiden.

Anneke Maissan worked as a nurse for 22 years, caring for parents and their children, at the Centre for Anthroposophical Health Care in Gouda. Since 1981, she has worked at the same place as a psycho-social worker, and is actively involved in biographical counselling, biographical courses and developmental issues.

From 1989 to 1998, **Paul Wormer** worked in Holland as an anthroposophical GP and school doctor. Between 1999 and 2006 he worked for Weleda, and at present works as a management consultant, specializing in health management for organizations, and as a vitality coach.

Preface

This book was written originally by a group of doctors and nurses, connected mostly with anthroposophical baby clinics in the Netherlands. First intended as a response to parents' questions about a more organic way of feeding their children, it was expanded to encompass the broad range of childcare advice given at these centres.

Written in 1994, the book is now in its sixth edition, and is used widely in the Netherlands and other countries. In 1999, a Dutch scientific study (the KOALA study) was performed among 2800 children to investigate the influence of lifestyle factors (and thus childcare measures) on allergic conditions. Five hundred of these children had parents who followed a so-called 'alternative lifestyle,' using more or less the childcare measures described in this book. The results of the KOALA study are published in this edition, showing that some of the advice described here has been shown to have a protective effect against allergic reactions.

Dr Marga Hogenboom has adapted the English version for instances where there are differences between the Dutch and British systems.

Machteld Huber, M.D.
Driebergen, 2008

The Baby Clinic

When a mother is expecting a child, this is the beginning of an exciting period; a time of 'expectation,' followed by the birth and the baby's first year. It is a special event every time, but particularly with a first child. Parenthood is 'born' along with the child, bringing all sorts of new tasks and experiences with it.

Baby clinics are located at health centres in virtually every town, and have the important task of monitoring the children and helping parents to look after their young children. In addition to ordinary baby clinics, there are also some clinics based on the approach used in anthroposophical medicine. In general, these are linked to anthroposophical medical practices.

All the work of these clinics is concerned with providing preventative care for children from birth to the age of four or five years. In general, this means providing help and support for parents to promote their child's health.

The doctor and nursing staff at the clinic devote their attention to the physical and psychological development of your child. They ask questions and examine the child to check for certain disorders: for example, growth or psychomotor disorders; disorders or malfunctions of the cardiovascular system, lungs, kidneys and reproductive organs; ear, nose and throat disorders; disorders of the abdomen, arms and legs; disorders of the teeth, and visual and hearing disorders.

At anthroposophical baby clinics, the constitutional characteristics of the child are also examined, and the personal characteristics and features, which might indicate a particular approach for medical and/or educational measures, are considered. After all, no child develops in accordance with the statistical norm. It is only by examining the individual developmental opportunities and problems of a child that it is possible to give appropriate advice. This is not so much a matter of preventing disorders, but of helping to ensure that the various developmental stages of the child follow each other in an appropriate way.

In addition, the baby clinic is an important place for parents to ask questions, as advice is offered on different subjects, including feeding and growth, upbringing and looking after the baby, physical and psychological development and the issue of inoculations.

The advice on children from birth to one year which you will find in this book is in line with the care provided by anthroposophical baby clinics, and may differ from the advice given by ordinary clinics, and is related to the views held by the doctor and nursing staff regarding the developing child. In Chapter 2 of this book you will find the viewpoints which form the background for the practical advice. This may be helpful when you want to make your own decision in a particular situation. However, this book serves to supplement rather than replace the supervision of the baby clinic. Whichever clinic you choose, it is important that you discuss any concerns you have, and express what you want, at the clinic.

We hope that the various subjects discussed will encourage a conscious approach to parenting and be helpful with regard to understanding, and living with, a developing child.

1. Pregnancy, Birth and Parenthood

Pregnancy

During pregnancy, the mother-to-be is in a very special condition, both physically and psychologically. There are all sorts of indications of a reduction in her level of consciousness, which may be manifested by drowsiness, diminished powers of concentration, dizziness, light-headedness and a floating sensation. At a physical level, there is a loss of muscular strength and a loss of tension in all the involuntary muscles. For example, the intestines work less effectively, which can result in constipation. There may also be changes in the action of the kidneys, blood pressure and pulse.

In a way, this whole condition resembles sleep. You could say that a pregnant woman floats between a waking and sleeping state and feels dreamier than she did before. Nevertheless, many women feel very well and active at the same time.

Pregnancy can be divided into three terms, each of roughly three months' duration.

In the first three months, the woman's organism has to be 'transformed' into a pregnant condition, or, as described above, the organism has to achieve a state between waking and sleeping. The fact that this is an intensive change is clear from the fact that the first three months of pregnancy are usually accompanied by nausea, vomiting and tiredness. It is during these months that the egg is fertilized, becomes embedded in the womb and the foetus starts to develop. It is a relatively vulnerable period of pregnancy in which miscarriages are fairly common (10%). See p.102 folic acid.

The second three-month term is usually the easiest. The pregnant woman becomes used to her condition, can do all sorts of things and does not experience much physical discomfort from the foetus. The foetus has become 'firmly established,' as is shown by the small number of problems during this period.

During the third stage, the physical manifestation of the child becomes increasingly clear, with a large stomach being the first sign of this. The discomfort which a pregnant woman experiences when bending down, urinating, feeling full after a meal, being unable to move, run, laugh and sit, reveals that the child has a clear physical presence. The foetus now becomes more vulnerable again. There may be bleeding or even a premature birth. At the end of this period, birth is often experienced as a real release.

When the woman has given birth, all the symptoms of the condition between waking and sleeping gradually disappear again. Only if she breastfeeds will this process be slightly postponed.

An overview of pregnancy reveals that the pregnant woman achieves a condition where she 'makes way' for the child to come; in which the child establishes a place on the way to birth. In a way, the expectant mother becomes less 'earthly,' while the child becomes increasingly 'earthbound.' From this perspective it is, therefore, not surprising that expectant mothers experience moments of contact with their unborn child. After all, both are in an 'interim state;' a state between the earthly world and the world that the child is coming from.

If we try to approach the woman's pregnancy in this manner — taking the idea of 'making way' seriously — it is clearly understandable that during pregnancy a woman often finds it difficult to tolerate direct confrontation with the world around her, and even tries to avoid it altogether. 'Listening' to her inner self is the best guideline.

It obviously goes without saying that alcohol and smoking should be avoided because they are known to affect the development and growth of the unborn child, and medicines should only be taken after consultation with the doctor. In addition, a natural, healthy and varied diet is clearly important for both mother and child.

To prepare for breastfeeding, it is a good idea to apply Weleda iris jelly to the nipples every day to prevent the skin cracking during breastfeeding. Stretch marks are largely dependant on genetic factors. However, it makes sense to keep the skin, particularly around the stomach and thighs, supple during pregnancy, by rubbing the skin twice daily with Weleda arnica massage oil. If there is a sensitivity to arnica, it is possible to use Weleda calendula massage oil.

The birth

Experiencing the birth of a child is one of the most intimate experiences in life. Feelings of astonishment, joy, anxiety, fear and fulfilment are experienced to extremes during the birth. Obviously these are most intense for the woman who is having the baby, but the family members and obstetric staff attending her fully share in the intensity of feeling.

It starts with the excitement and anticipation of what will happen when the waters break or the first contractions start. Getting everything ready, the support and help of the midwife during contractions, the constant question of how far the process has advanced — these are all part of the active and busy atmosphere of birth. However, sometimes there are also moments of near serenity and tranquillity; an atmosphere of relaxation, trust and complete surrender to what is to come.

The birth takes place in these recurrent and alternating periods of intense activity and intense tranquillity. Everyone attending the birth finds that a unique atmosphere develops as a result of these alternate emotions, which can go on for many hours. It is an incomparable atmosphere, evoking feelings of deep wonder and awe.

The focal point of everything that is going on is the mother-to-be. She is in touch with the deepest natural forces in her body, and is in danger of being overwhelmed by these natural forces, with an intensity which rarely occurs in life. She may also feel that she does not have the strength to give birth on her own, and may be very grateful to accept the instructions of the obstetric staff, so that the sense of impotence can make way for a sense of trust in the successful end of the birth.

When the cervix is fully dilated, the moment arrives when she can use all her strength to help the child to be born by pushing it out. Just before this moment, it is quite common for the woman's consciousness to be almost overwhelmed, and then return quite vivdly with the first push. This stage of pushing the baby out is extremely hard work, even though sometimes it only requires one big contraction.

From the moment that the baby's head emerges, the atmosphere changes immediately. All attention is focused on the delivery of the rest of the baby, who eventually experiences light, air and gravity for the first time, is placed on its mother's stomach and swaddled in warm nappies (diapers). If not giving birth at home, you should check with your midwife or consultant to see if it is possible to have a warm cloth to swaddle the baby in. All eyes are on the baby; the noises, movements, eyes and hair. Everyone feels an urge to touch the baby and stroke it.

Then the obstetrician focuses on the last part of the delivery: cutting the umbilical cord and delivering the placenta.

The whole birth is only really complete when the mother has been washed and cleaned up, and is holding the pink, warm, swaddled baby in her arms, and is surrounded by everyone who was present at the birth. The whole spectrum of emotions is experienced, together with a sense of satisfaction, gratitude and respect for the forces that play a role in the birth process.

The birth described above is probably the birth every parent dreams of. And yet, no two births are the same. The life of every person starts with a unique event; the delivery. Some children have a difficult start, for example, if the birth was induced too early, the baby was born prematurely, or if the delivery involved a great deal of medical intervention. In the UK most babies are now born in hospital, but it is possible to discuss your birth plan beforehand with your midwife or consultant.

For parents, the fear about the baby's health or being overwhelmed by a premature birth can obstruct the feelings of wonder and gratitude described above. Sometimes it may be a while before you can start to love your child in a relaxed way and feel an obvious connection with it, particularly if you feel unsure or anxious. This takes time, so you must try and take the time that is needed. If you were admitted to hospital, you can organize a sort of second birth experience, so that when the baby comes home, you can get used to each other, feel each other, and build up a new life together. Many parents have described that this helped them to recognise the healthy aspects of the child and his lust for life.

Parenthood

The birth of a child is an intense experience for the parents, particularly the birth of their first child. In fact, it brings about many changes. Before the birth the parents had a relationship with each other, and after the birth they have suddenly become parents and formed a family. Obviously, they still have a relationship, but the partners no longer relate exclusively to each other. In particular, the mother focuses body and soul on her child. After the birth it may be a very long time, sometimes as long as a year, before she feels her old self. Consequently, owing to the new situation in which they find themselves, parents have to redefine the way in which they relate to each other.

This process is extremely demanding because the father and mother are involved with the child in very different ways during pregnancy and birth, and during the initial period after birth. The father may have a tendency to continue his old life with some modifications, while the mother has a deep sense that everything has changed. It may be a while before the partners find a new way of relating to each other on the basis of these two different worlds of experience. It is important to take time for this process and talk about it together from time to time.

What was described above applies particularly for the situation in which mother, father and child(ren) form the family. Where there is a one-parent family from birth, this process will particularly concern the mother.

After the birth, another process starts as well in that all parents discover themselves in a new way. They experience new positive feelings, although they can also have a negative character. A child brings happiness and joy, but there are also moments when irritation reaches unimagined heights.

In the whole range of emotions evoked by a child, feelings of anxiety have a special place, giving rise to questions such as: Am I doing it right? Will anything happen to my child or me? Will everything be okay?

Every step in the child's development is another step out into the world. From the age of three, the child even ventures beyond the horizons of the parents; he walks around the block or goes to school for the first time.

Some people are more sensitive to these anxieties than others, but since this anxiety is fruitless — and can really make life difficult for a child — something should be found to counterbalance it. Sometimes gaining an insight into the situation helps to diminish the anxiety, but often this is not enough. In order to tackle the anxiety in a structured way, it may be necessary to work on strengthening the parents' confidence. Obviously this does not mean blind faith that 'everything will probably be alright.' It is not as simple as that. It means that it is possible to work on the confidence about the direction in which the child is moving, even though unexpected and undesired events may play a role. While anxiety is often 'our own problem,' confidence can become a strength, which allows the child to flourish; having confidence in someone gives them the strength to grow.

In addition, a child often gives us a new sense of self-awareness: with his behaviour and imitations, he holds up a mirror to his parents. From the age of a few months you will see that a child assimilates the world by imitating it. The child copies everything he encounters, both internally and externally. For parents, this means that *what* they do and *how* they do things is important. Whether we do things hastily or with care, whether we do things unwillingly or with joy; all these aspects permeate the actions we perform and are unconsciously assimilated and imitated by the child. This also applies to what we say. Long before the child can understand our words, he will be aware of our intentions. Experiencing this, and occasionally having the things which we do and say, and how we do and say them, reflected by a child will lead to self-awareness, and possibly to a change in our way of being and doing things.

In positive terms, a child stimulates us to develop ourselves as well. There is also a third process. By experiencing the development of a small child and feeling co-responsible for him, it is possible to focus on your own childhood. Some things from your own childhood can lead to the feeling that 'I want to do things for my children like that as well,' while at other moments, you feel that 'I want to spare my children this or that.' Sometimes this encounter with your own past can be quite intense. It's good to know that it is not unusual.

Just as we re-examine our own past, we also start to have a different view of the future; in a sense looking to the future through the child. The future shines through the small child and urges us to determine the structure for that future.

Above, we have highlighted a number of the issues which will confront every parent; the redefinition of the relationship with their partner and other members of the family, a re-definition of themselves, and a new view of the past and the future.

2. General Points of View

In this section we describe a number of points of view which serve as a guideline for the way we view, and relate to, young children.

The child's development and care, sleeping and waking, play and toys, safety and feeding are subjects which will be tackled in this section in terms of content. A practical approach to these subjects can be found under the advice for every stage (see Chapters 3–6).

The child's development

From the moment the child is born, the parents have the important task of monitoring his or her development. This gives rise to many questions. How can we best prepare for the child's future? Should we, or should we not, familiarize the child with elements of adult life at an early stage, so that she will be prepared for this later on? The answers to these questions will depend on your view of the child's developmental stages.

We proceed on the assumption that the more successfully a child is able to fully develop at a particular stage, the more harmonious the development will be. This also applies for future development.

For a baby and young child, this means that we must create the conditions in which a baby can most successfully be a baby, and a young child can most successfully be a young child.

The first developmental stage after birth is strongly centred on the child's physical and motor development. Growth is quite exceptional during the first year of life, and is still rather like the growth of the embryo. The development and growth, which takes place outside the womb in humans, takes place completely inside the womb in other mammals. When the child is one year old, the development has reached a level comparable to the birth level of other mammals.

For the baby's development, it is good if the conditions after birth are still quite similar to the situation in the womb. This particularly concerns the protective cocoon around the child. Warmth, a sense of security and some protection against environmental influences promote the baby's health. It is extremely important for the baby's physical development for her to have physical contact — rocking, cuddling or simply holding the baby in your arms. Children who lack this physical contact do not develop well, even if they have 'the best feeding.' These babies immediately start to grow again when attention and care is devoted to physical contact. Satisfying the need for physical contact gives the child a basis for the rest of his or her life.

Nevertheless, in humans, a good environment alone does not guarantee development. Every person has his own rate of development and his own way of developing. For example, there are babies who develop motor skills very quickly, sit up at an early stage, roll over, stand and walk. On the other hand, other children appear to 'stand still' in their development for a long time, then seem to miss out a few stages and can suddenly walk, even though they never crawled. Some children start to develop speech very early, while others remain unintelligible for a long time.

It is important to be aware of a child's own way of developing. There may be a tendency to a certain one-sidedness. This sort of one-sidedness — for example, the slow development of speech — can be regarded as the child's own way of developing. It is only when this one-sidedness is particularly strong that it may be seen as a developmental disorder.

Thus, the first year of the child's development can be seen as a continuation of the embryonic stage.

During this first year of life, the body matures to the extent that the child becomes able to control it for herself. A one-year-old child can stand and go where she likes and move about freely in space. It is as though she is taking charge of her own physical body. This stage of development depends on healthy physical growth and development. Illness and malnutrition will immediately delay the process. Development at this stage is mainly influenced by the physical organism and the care of this organism.

The basis for the later development of speech is laid during the first year of life. Talk to, and with, the baby, and play with her. She sees the gestures which accompany words, and hears the songs. All this contributes to the child becoming increasingly familiar with human language. The clearest sign of this is contented *baby talk* by the end of the first year of life.

After the first year, the child depends on being able to imitate what she has heard. She will start to copy the words herself, first words of one syllable and then words of several syllables. She then begins to combine words, and finally produces short sentences. In this way, the child enters a second area in which she can move about freely — the field of language. By mastering speech and language, the child takes part in social life in her own way, and becomes able to express herself through the spoken word.

The next stage of development is the time at which the child starts to say 'I.' Prior to that stage the child called herself by her own name. This can be seen as an expression of the fact that the child was not yet deeply connected with her own body; thus in a sense the child saw herself from outside, as other people see her.

When she becomes more closely connected with her own body, the first, still primitive, sense of self-consciousness emerges and the child experiences a sense of self; she starts to say 'I' and experiences herself as a centre. As a result of this process, the child may also feel cut off from the world around her.

By the age of three or four, the child has gone through a sort of first cycle of development. By learning to stand and walk, she has achieved a certain degree of freedom in space. By learning to speak and understand, she can develop socially and communicate with others. With the deeper connection of the self and the body, self-consciousness emerges for the first time, and this is expressed when the child uses the word 'I' to talk about herself.

Learning to use language independently is an important psychological development, as is developing a sense of individuality. However, healthy physical development is always a prerequisite for this. Motor development is particularly important for the development of psychological functions later on. Playing with bricks, simple ball games, finger games, circle games — in short, everything we do with the physical organism of the child as the point of contact — will have a positive influence on development.

The behaviour of the people in the child's direct environment is very important for development. A small child learns and develops by imitating what she sees, hears, feels and so on. In this way the child learns to walk, speak and think, and during this first learning process carefully assimilates all the details — particularly during the first three years. This once again underlines the importance of being conscious of our own behaviour as well as the material environment of the child (see also Impressions, p.25).

Admittedly, the aspects of child development described here are very general, but they can still provide a direction for the way in which we behave with the child. The care for the physical processes of growth and development are of central importance. We can measure and weigh growth, while we can assess development from the development of the motor system, the mastery of language, and the birth of the 'self' when the child starts to say 'I'.

Sleeping and waking

During the course of life a person's need for sleep undergoes great changes. A newborn baby often sleeps for between eighteen and twenty hours out of every twenty-four. A one-year-old can sleep for fourteen hours, while an adult needs between six and eight hours of sleep. Therefore, in the first year of life, the child should spend a great deal of the time asleep.

We have seen that there are two important things in this first year — growth (a baby's weight triples in the first year) and development. Growth takes place particularly during sleep, while development is stimulated during the waking hours. The various organs 'learn' to operate in a sense, with the use of the body during the daytime (by eating, moving, etc.). What the organs 'learn' during the day continues to have an effect while the baby sleeps, and is assimilated in the body's growth activity.

A one-sided predominance of growth and excessive stimulation to develop both have a negative effect. There should be a healthy balance between the two processes; an alternation between waking and sleeping which is suitable for each stage. When the child is about one year old, this balance will have become established in the operation of the organs, in a particular day/night rhythm — the biological clock.

For good health and for the child to be able to make use of his physical capabilities properly, it is essential for this day/night rhythm to become well established. Therefore, it is literally of vital importance for a small child to establish a steady pattern during the day with regard to sleeping, eating and waking.

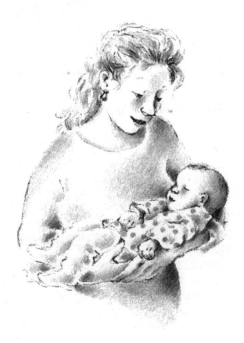

A steady pattern of set times in the life of a child promotes growth and development and helps to establish a healthy rhythm of sleeping and waking. Too much stimulation during the day may prevent the child from falling asleep; however, a completely *unstimulating* environment, without healthy challenges for the child, can also lead to problems with sleep because the child is not sufficiently tired. A healthy routine in the day, alternating challenges and periods of quiet, being together and being alone, can help to correct sleeping problems. Rituals for going to sleep can also be helpful — rocking, singing lullabies, the use of musical boxes or a prayer for the child are methods used by many families.

Sleeping well means that the child must be able to surrender and 'let go.' This is not as easy for some children as for others. It is helpful to give the child a sense of security, for example, in the enclosed space of the cradle (possibly with a hood) or lying against the mother. Warmth promotes a sense of comfort and relaxation; a bonnet, a sleeping bag, some drops of lavender water on the pillow, or a hot water bottle can sometimes help babies who find it difficult to fall asleep. Hot water bottles should always be removed *before* the baby is placed in the warm cradle. A light silk bonnet is appropriate for indoor use, but be aware of the risk of overheating. Wrapping the child up firmly provides a sense of security as well as a feeling of warmth.

However, there are babies who assimilate everything that happens around them so greedily that they actively seem to suppress their feelings of tiredness and the need for sleep. The more stimulation they are given, the hungrier they seem to be. They are unable to set their own boundaries. Increasingly, we see babies who spend many hours of the day — and sometimes the night — awake, constantly asking for attention from the environment. For these children, the parents must learn to see when they show signs of being sleepy. The fact that this is quite an art is clear from the many stories told about this problem. If you miss the right moment, the child appears to go past his sleepiness and will keep going for many hours. Signs of sleepiness are restlessness or agitation, looking away, rubbing the eyes and face, warm hands and red ears, grizzling and crying. By responding to these signs of sleep immediately and consistently, by placing the baby in his cot, it is possible to create a healthy need for sleep. By not responding straightaway every time the baby cries, he will learn to resolve minor discomfort for himself. It is important to realize that any attention wakes the baby up. All the extra attention and special behaviour associated with going to sleep often achieve quite the opposite of what the parents hope to achieve.

Care

Boundaries

Birth is an immense change for the baby. Her whole physiology changes fundamentally and she experiences a completely new environment. The boundaries of the womb are left behind and she enters a 'boundless' world. In the womb, the child was able to grow harmoniously, protected from the world.

This reveals that everything that is developing requires a protective environment. With a newborn baby, and actually throughout childhood, this protective environment is constantly provided to establish firm foundations for later life. Unconsciously, the child is constantly reminded of the situation in the womb, which is related to an experience of security, safety, protection and fundamental confidence.

Warmth

The womb not only protects the embryo from the world; it also surrounds it with an even temperature of 37°C (98.6°F). A 'warm environment' is provided in the best possible way.

After birth, a child has to learn to maintain her own body temperature at a constant level, at first with the help of adults. She must interrelate the warm and cold parts of the body. This is achieved by means of a sensitive metabolic process which generates heat.

Normal growth and the development of the normal physical processes are also dependent on this metabolism. All the heat which the baby does not have to produce herself in order to maintain her temperature at the right level will benefit growth.

It takes the child a long time to regulate her own temperature; the normal difference of 1°C (2°F). between the body temperature during the night and the day is achieved by most children between their fifth and ninth months. Up to that time they are extremely dependent on the extra warmth provided in the form of good physical care, clothes, and hot water bottles used to warm the cradle *before* they are placed in it.

The ability to distinguish whether something is hot or cold is learnt during the initial period. The better this ability has been developed by providing sufficient warmth in childhood, the better the child can use it at a later age.

Cold feet are an important sign that extra attention should be devoted to regulating the child's temperature. A baby should have warm feet, warm legs, a warm body and warm arms.

Special attention to warmth also has another significance. A warm environment helps the child to 'warm up' for life on earth. However, our motto is not 'the warmer, the better,' because always being dressed in too many clothes or being covered up can actually make a child either drowsy or very restless, and overheating can be very dangerous. Detailed research has revealed that there is a relationship between overheating and cot death. Duvets and synthetic materials can especially cause overheating. Therefore we certainly advise against using these.

In our view, the important thing is to learn to observe the needs of the child with regard to warmth, and to read the signs when more or less warmth needs to be provided in the form of clothes, bedding or ambient heating. The body temperature of the child is the most important thermometer, and in a healthy baby, this fluctuates around 37°C (98.6°F). You can learn to take the baby's temperature with your hands so that you can literally feel how the child is regulating its own temperature. In the first week or two after birth, take the baby's temperature every day, as well as feeling how warm she is. Then start testing yourself: feel how warm the baby is, then predict her temperature and check with the thermometer for a few days. If your predictions are correct, you will only have to take the baby's temperature when you are doubtful or if she is sick.

Impressions

Everything we do, feel and think around the child is assimilated by the child. She is still completely open and has a boundless trust in the environment. The buffer which we have between ourselves and the world as adults is formed by recognising and understanding that world. A small child is not yet able to do this. Up to about the third year, the child identifies with the environment in which she is living in a very natural way. This is followed by a stage in which thinking gradually assumes set patterns, and the child leans to distinguish herself from the outside world. For the first time, she makes a distinction between her own individuality and the world which is perceived. In this light it is understandable that first memories only go back to the third year, and there are no, or very few, memories before this.

The child is one big sensory organ. Up to the third year, all impressions are assimilated in an uninhibited way and disappear into the subconscious. There they are combined with other physical processes, and a sort of *print* is made; it is as though the child models the influences of the environment in its own 'clay.' Therefore, it is important that we are aware of what 'goes into' the child — also for later on.

Example. *A child in a boat on the water, experiences the swell, feels the sunlight on her skin and the wind in her hair, smells the odour of water and fish, is taking in healthy impressions which build up the whole organism. The situation is quite different for a child at a* *department store who is placed in a rotating ship, which goes round and round when a coin is placed in the machine. The child will enjoy both these experiences, but they affect the organism in significantly different ways. The 'boat on the water' situation sounds idyllic; this is usually a vacation experience. However, there are also impressions closer to home, which can be constructive and have the above-mentioned character.*

Positive, constructive impressions are those impressions in which the natural origin of materials, sounds etc, can be perceived by the child. For hearing, these are the sounds of people and animals, and natural sounds such as the rustling of the wind. For sight, they are natural colours. For the sense of touch, they are materials such as wool, cotton, silk, wood, sand and water.

Many domestic appliances such as vacuum cleaners, washing machines, radio, television and plastic toys were created as a result of human technical ingenuity. For children, these are actually an abstraction, lacking in natural connection.

Radio, television and plastic toys are things you can consciously choose to have or not to have in a small child's immediate environment. With household appliances, you can take care to minimize the sound in the baby's immediate environment. So-called 'white noise'

from household appliances is not a good idea for the young child as it blocks out normal impressions. Autistic children can also become obsessed by white noise. Playing a lyre, humming or singing are better background sounds for the child.

Simple actions such as washing hands, or sweeping up with a dustpan and brush in the child's presence show how things are done. These actions are enjoyable and you can invite children to imitate them.

The feelings of people around the child also have an effect. It is obvious that a child will thrive best in a genuine atmosphere of joy and warmth. This has a positive effect. But there is not a parent in the world that is always cheerful and relaxed at every moment of the day (and night). It is worth aiming to achieve these qualities, but at times when you do not succeed, you must take them for what they are — also real human emotions. In every family there are days when everything goes pear-shaped and the ideal image of a happy family seems a long way off. Humour is always a good remedy. It can be a relief if you can laugh about yourself and the situation.

The needs which were mentioned above — that is, the need for boundaries, warmth and positive impressions — make great demands on the environment. It means that parents must have clear insight and a good level of empathy to get things right: too cold or too warm, too many impressions or too quiet, well-protected or not enough room to breathe?

From this point of view, we would like to discuss a number of practical aspects of childcare.

Clothes

Clothes are like a second skin, which support the functions of the skin. The skin helps to regulate body temperature and protects us from infections. In addition, the skin is a sensory organ with which we perceive the environment. These three functions are most effectively supported with clothes made of wool, silk, cotton or hemp. These fibres are preferable as they provide sense impressions from a natural source via the skin, which help the child to build up its body. Other fibres are more alien, and even viscose, which is made from cotton or wood, is processed quite strongly, in a way which is now known to be quite polluting.

Wool

Sheep's wool protects the sheep from heat and cold, rain and toxic waste. The curls trap the warm air around the sheep's skin. The wool keeps out the rain, and waste products are absorbed and emitted through the wool via perspiration.

All these qualities are found in woollen clothes. The warmth of the wool protects the child from cooling down too quickly and supports her unstable heat regulation system which cannot yet retain body heat.

Its absorbent capacity (30 to 40%) ensures that the child remains comfortably dry. The quality of the wool depends on the age of the sheep, the animal's diet and health, as well as the way in which the wool was turned into clothing.

Finely knitted woollen vests are available, which form a soft, flexible outer skin. Woollen jumpers and cardigans should be loose fitting so that they are easy to put on and take off. Woollen pants are wonderful to use over cotton nappies. They can be knitted easily, preferably from slightly greasy sheep's wool, and are ideal for absorbing moisture and neutralizing the waste products in urine.

A woollen shawl will keep the baby warm when there are fluctuations in temperature. Woollen socks will also keep the feet nice and warm. Furthermore, wool does not attract dirt, and therefore woollen clothes do not have to washed as often as cotton clothes, though they do have to be aired regularly.

Silk

The silkworm spins its cocoon of silk thread, in which the worm is sealed off from any negative external influences. The silk is made under the influence of sunlight — at sunset, the silkworm stops spinning, and at sunrise, it starts work again.

If you use silk in clothes, you will feel its enclosing qualities. Furthermore, silk can absorb 30% of its weight in moisture without feeling damp. In addition, silk retains heat when it is cold and releases heat when it is warm. That is why silk is worn especially in summer. Silk and, in particular, knitted silk is an excellent basic material for vests, but it is advisable to put a woollen vest over the silk vest as well.

Children who are sensitive to wool against the skin, and children who are very sensitive to impressions and consequently become restless, will benefit from wearing a silk vest.

Cotton

Cotton is widely used nowadays for children's clothes, especially as this material can be washed so easily in the washing machine. At the same time, it should be said that it actually has to be washed often because it attracts dirt easily. Cotton can absorb 20% of its own weight in moisture.

As cotton cannot absorb heat, this passes easily through the material to the outside air. Consequently, this material is not the best choice for a child's underclothes throughout the year. Furthermore, the way in which cotton is grown is not particularly environmentally friendly, and chemical products are often used in the treatment of the material. Fortunately, there are several eco-cotton projects which now promote its environmentally-friendly cultivation and processing, and eco-cotton is becoming increasingly available in shops and over the internet.

We suggest dressing the baby in at least two layers of clothing, covering the whole body, including the arms, legs and feet. This produces a layer of air between the two layers which retains heat. In a temperate climate, a long-sleeved woollen vest — or a vest of wool and silk — can be worn for most of the year.

In practice, we regularly find that babies are not dressed warmly enough, and they are often restless and troubled by stomach cramps, or they are constantly crying. The simple remedy of dressing the child more warmly, in better fitting clothes, will do wonders for this.

Bonnets

Unfortunately, bonnets are no longer in fashion. In comparison with the rest of their bodies, little babies often have an enormous — and sometimes rather bald — head. The head is constantly losing heat, which should really be retained for the development of the brain and organs. On the one hand, a silk bonnet will retain the baby's heat, and on the other hand, it protects the head and the open fontanel from a restless environment. It is important for the forehead to be free, because this part of the body acts as a sort of thermostat for regulating body heat. Where it is often windy, it may also be necessary for the baby to wear a second bonnet made of wool. There are wonderful bonnets on sale, or they can be knitted in material which is so soft that it is like a second skin.

Bonnets can be removed when the child is in the cot as long as the baby is well protected.

Wraps and swaddling

Because of the need for boundaries, it is understandable why many babies, as well as older children, calm down and fall asleep easily when they are firmly tucked in, or if they are wrapped up or swaddled.

Usually, babies have a flannel sheet wrapped around them, during the postnatal period, but this often disappears, to be replaced by a baby-gro/sleepsuit. We recommend continuing to use a swaddling cloth and wrapping it firmly around the baby-gro/sleepsuit before putting the baby to bed (see illustration). As the baby still lies with its arms and legs bent, it should be swaddled in this position, to increase the sense of security. The baby can now relax and will fall asleep warm and snug. However, you must make sure that the baby is not wrapped up too warmly (see p.25).

The woollen wrap can serve as a blanket outside the cot for when the baby is fed. When the woollen cloth is no longer sufficient, use a (woollen) baby sleeping bag for in bed.

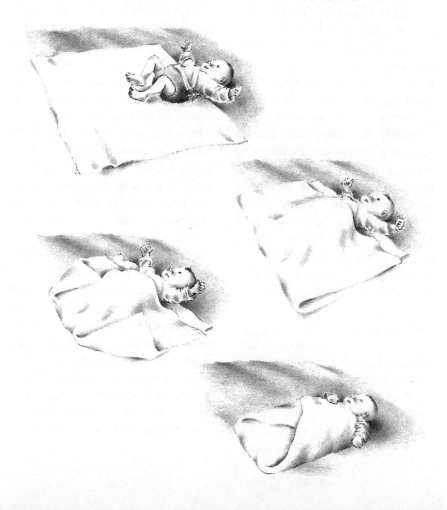

Children who remain restless and have difficulty falling asleep despite being wrapped up, as well as babies who do not establish a good rhythm of drinking/sleeping, may benefit from the old-fashioned method of swaddling in which the arms are also wrapped up so that the child cannot flail about. Flailing is often a response to crying, cramps or fright, but because it is involuntary, it can cause new restlessness. Swaddling can help to break this vicious circle.

Many parents find it difficult to restrict their baby in this way; in our age of boundless freedom, it is not so easily accepted. However, parents usually overcome their resistance when they see how the baby responds to swaddling. For most babies, it results in a much greater sense of peace, and consequently they sleep well and establish a pattern of sleeping and feeding every few hours. Nowadays, two methods of swaddling are recommended: either ready-made swaddling blankets or swaddling wraps, or using the method shown at the back of this book (see p.108). (See also Blom, *Crying and Restlessness in Babies*.)

The cradle

The cradle is an important successor of the smallest home in which the baby lived before birth. You can opt for a basket cradle (Moses basket), a wooden (rocking) cradle or a cot. For safety considerations, the baby's feet should always be placed at the end of a cot, with its head halfway down. Tuck in the blanket in such a way that the head is free and the shoulders are covered. A hood or canopy over the cradle or cot makes the space more intimate, so that the child is not distracted by the environment and can sleep more peacefully.

For the canopy, it is best to use plain materials in soft colours. A canopy made of light blue silk combined with a layer of pink silk gives a very subtle calming colour.

The mattress must be absolutely flat, providing good support, and it must be well-ventilated and warm. Our preference is for a mattress of kapok, cotton or another natural material. A sheep's fleece can be placed on the mattress. The fleece is soft and gives a beneficial warmth so that the newborn baby is protected from cooling down too quickly. Make sure that the fleece is not too large and lies on the mattress without any folds. Cover the fleece with a sheet. The bedding should be made of cotton and wool. Do not use synthetic materials. The sheets and blankets should be big enough to tuck the baby in quite firmly. The fleece and the mattress should be regularly aired. If you use a woollen wrap there are likely to be patches of damp under the mattress. If necessary, use a waterproof sheet. There are cotton sheets available that are impregnated with rubber and do not

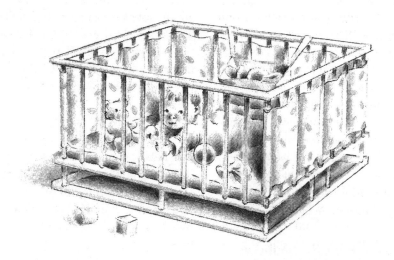

feel clammy. We do not recommend the use of duvets, even those made of wool, because of the risk of suffocation.

If the cradle is next to the window, watch out for overheating in the sun. A baby can easily become too hot in a heated room when the sun shines through the window.

The playpen

Up to the age of four months, it is not really necessary to have a playpen. Nevertheless, when the baby is downstairs, it is a good idea to have a safe place to place it. A wicker basket with a soft cover, or the bed of a pram, are quite suitable.

We do not recommend the frequent use of a *baby seat* or *recliner,* as the baby is stimulated by the ac-

tion of sitting in an upright position at a stage when he is still physically immature. The baby can only lie passively in a *baby seat,* which does not matter for a short period, but is harmful to physical development in the long term.

This objection does not apply so much to the use of a recliner, but there are other objections; when the baby discovers that he can bounce the recliner with one leg, he often finds it difficult to stop, even when he gets tired of the mechanical movement.

When the baby starts to reach out for things and becomes more active in its motor development, it is time for a playpen. Quite apart from the fact that this provides a safe place for the child to learn to sit and stand, it is often a favourite place for being quiet and for playing undisturbed. A cloth cover, like a curtain, along three sides of the playpen will increase the sense of security, and is not to be confused with cot bumpers, which are not recommended as they pose a suffocation risk for the young child. For motor development, it is important that the floor of the playpen is sturdy and not too smooth (for example, a cloth folded double), so that the child can roll over and can put pressure on it.

Walkers and baby bouncers

We emphatically advise *against* the use of walkers and baby bouncers. These are 'aids' which speed up the child's motor development in an unnatural way. Children certainly like to use these things — especially if they can move around in them quickly — and want to use them more and more. However, it is much better for a child to learn to stand and walk at his own pace. In this sense, walkers and baby bouncers do not help healthy development in any way, and are actually more of a deterrent to healthy development.

Prams and baby carriers (slings)

The pram can be a safe and sheltered place in which the baby can sleep outside during the first few months. For walking, a baby carrier is often a better alternative because it means that the baby moves in time with the pace at which the adult is walking, and is not shaken about so much as in a pram, as it goes up and down the pavement. The child is carried in a natural position in a baby carrier (sling), (see the illustration on p.106).

However, at this point a warning should be given. It has been shown that babies can become too hot and stuffy, particularly if carried under a coat. Unfortunately, there are even a few cases, which resulted in a baby's death. We recommend that you keep a careful eye on a baby in a baby carrier, and if possible carry it on top of a coat rather than underneath, with, if necessary, a woollen cloth around the baby.

The disadvantage of a baby carrier in which the baby is in a vertical position is that the baby did not take up this position itself. In this sense, the baby carrier is not for babies until they reach the age of nine months. A sling is preferable, as the whole back and head are supported, although it might be tiring for the mother to carry.

When a baby has reached the age for a pram, the best model is one in which the baby faces the parent. In this way, the baby constantly has the comforting face of its father or mother in front of it, and can find out from that face what is happening in the big wide world. A traditional pram has the advantage that the child lies flat, as at this age the baby's head is still relatively heavy and the neck cannot keep the head in a stable position. We recommend a buggy only from the age when the child is able to sit unassisted.

Toys and playing

A newborn baby has a special relationship with the world around it. In the first place, the child and his world are still one, and all the impressions from that world have a deep effect on the child's organism. This applies to the baby's food, but also for impressions, such as the arms rocking him or the sound of lullabies.

In addition, we find that everything the child does is a form of play. The whole voyage of discovery of his own body takes place with great perseverance, as well as with great joy. For example, the child sees and discovers his hands and puts them together. Although these are uncontrolled movements at first, the baby practises this hand-eye coordination time and time again. The pleasure he gets from this is quite tangible.

The baby needs very few toys during his first year, actually no more than what is available in the home in terms of safe and attractive shapes, and what you can make simply yourself. The fewer objects in the child's environment, the more thoroughly these will be explored, held, sucked and eventually understood. If the child has too many toys he cannot choose; attention to the world, interest and concentration can actually be practised best when the child has few objects around him.

Background music should also be avoided. It distracts the child from listening to the sounds produced by his own activities.

Every object should be simple and straightforward, so that it leaves something to the child's imagination.

We should focus our attention not only on the safety of the material, but also ask ourselves whether the child can gain different experiences. A piece of wood has a particular weight, which can be felt and a grain which can be examined with the fingertips. Both elements reveal very different things from a cuddly toy. The child's gaze can be captured by bright colours and rigid, caricatured shapes; his eyes are powerfully drawn to the object, and it is no longer possible to pay attention to it in a free and playful way. This applies to an extreme extent with regard to television.

It is a good idea to alternate playing alone and playing together. On the one hand, it is good for the child's development to learn to play alone and experience things in a quiet, peaceful atmosphere. On the other hand, the parent and child can gain a great deal of pleasure, for example, from playing games while the child sits on his parent's lap, giving and taking bricks and so on. The practical sections of this book explore further possibilities in greater detail.

Play is an essential element in a child's life. It is a preparation for being able to work with concentration and enthusiasm in adult life.

Safety

The child's safety is an important part of upbringing. Parents can avoid many dangerous situations, though not all, by taking *safety measures* in and around the house.

Keeping an eye on the child, knowing where he is and what he is doing, is the second important factor with regard to safety at home.

The third factor is concerned with *teaching* the child. You can teach your child safe behaviour by helping him to learn to recognise dangerous situations, by teaching all sorts of skills properly (going up and down stairs, cycling etc.) and by insisting on obedience, particularly with regard to safety. This third factor, teaching safety, hardly plays any role during the first year. Safety measures in and around the house are discussed in the practical section of the book (see Chapters 3–6).

Many children learn to do something new at a time when you are not really expecting it. Suddenly they appear to be able to roll over or stand up in their cot. Anticipate these situations and make sure that you take the right safety precautions in good time. The description of successive psychomotor skills may help in this respect.

Parents' behaviour also contributes to making the environment more or less safe. Clear discipline in the home, clear habits and customs, a good safety routine and clear agreements — also with brothers and sisters — will increase safety. Nevertheless, it is an art to remember these, even in unexpected situations (the telephone ringing, unexpected visits etc).

Keeping an eye on the child in the first few months mainly means not leaving the baby alone on the dressing table or wherever you change his nappies, and knowing whether there are any brothers, sisters or pets near him. From the moment that the baby starts to crawl, stand and walk, it becomes increasingly important to keep an eye on him, because the area in which he moves becomes larger and larger.

Feeding

A person has to eat and drink every day to live. Food is a fundamental, and if all is well, a joyful aspect of life, particularly in the first few years of life. In fact, the child has to learn to digest, step by step. The digestive system develops as a result of digesting food. The importance of feeding the baby becomes particularly clear when she is very small: she meets the world and relates to it in such a way that the food is assimilated and incorporated as her own substance.

The quality of food and feeding

The child has a natural propensity for learning to digest all sorts of natural products. If there is not enough time for this learning process, if the preparation is not adapted to the age of the child, or if, for example, unnatural substances — such as colouring agents or taste enhancers — are added to the food, the digestive process may become disrupted, giving rise to problems. One example of this is over-sensitivity to food. Fortunately, many problems can be resolved, but it is best to use as few products with artificial additives as possible in the baby's food.

Another aspect is the nutritional quality of the products themselves. These days everyone knows about calories and carbohydrates, proteins and fats, and it is easy to forget that our food consists of substances that were originally alive.

The quality of the food is related not only to the composition of a product, but also to its vitality. This in turn relates to the way in which the living product was able to grow and develop. Vitality does not thrive when the process is hurried, and the vitality of a food crop also flourishes best when there is harmonious development with no artificial fertilizers to accelerate growth. Harmonious development also means that crops are less susceptible to disease and infestation, so that fewer insecticides and weed-killers have to be used.

Products, which are grown biodynamically or organically, comply with these conditions of cultivation. In addition, these types of farming devote a great deal of attention to promoting the vitality of the soil and crops. Therefore, organically and biodynamically (often marked Demeter) grown products are preferable for the baby's diet. These kinds of products are usually sold in health food shops.

The advice on feeding given below reveals that a great deal of attention is devoted to cereals. In western food habits, potatoes as well as meat have an important place. However, a diet consisting of different cereals, such as rice, millet, oats and buckwheat (which is actually not a cereal), when supplemented with dairy products, constitutes just as balanced a diet as potatoes and meat. In fact, our preference is for cereals, because they are harmonious food crops, strongly related to light and the warmth of the sun, which are extremely important factors for nutrition. Cereals are also preferable from the point of view of the environment, because their cultivation is relatively less harmful than the cultivation of potatoes.

In our opinion, a balanced diet should consist of cereals combined with dairy products, nuts, fresh fruit and vegetables, all grown biodynamically or organically. Obviously, a small child gradually develops to include these in her diet, and the following guidelines may prove useful. Peanuts should be avoided with children with a family history of atopia (allergy) until the age of three years. Other nuts should be avoided where the child is known to react to peanuts.

At the baby clinic, advice on feeding is related to the individual child as well as the wishes and possibilities of the parents. After all, eating should be a pleasure. Healthy digestion is promoted by a pleasure in food and by eating in a relaxed and friendly atmosphere.

The development of feeding

The development of a child in her first year is enormous. In the space of just one year, she develops from a sleeping baby lying in her cot to a toddler, fully alert, standing in her playpen. This development is reflected in the development of feeding.

Initially eating and drinking are one — all the food is liquid and absorbed by means of *breastfeeding* or *bottle-feeding*. During the course of the first six months, *solids* are added — puréed fruit and vegetables, given on a spoon. During the second six months, these solids become more varied and thicker by adding cereals. A bowl of porridge is also introduced to replace the breast or bottle-feeding.

By the end of the first year, the child is eating real food and drinking real drinks. Up to this point, vegetables have been puréed in a thick liquid form, but by now they are usually cut up into chunkier pieces. The child can eat her first sandwich and drink from a beaker. All this is quite different from the situation at the beginning.

Breastfeeding

If at all possible, we always advise breastfeeding for the first few months, even if the mother goes back to work and can only breastfeed for a short time. In view of the great advantages of breastfeeding, the baby will profit from any mother's milk it can get. For example, the milk produced for the first few days after birth, the so-called *colostrum,* cannot be matched by any type of bottle-feeding because of its wealth of antibodies and vitamins.

During the following months, breast milk also continues to protect the baby from infections. Breastfeeding provides the most suitable food for the digestive organs of the child, which are still developing. Breastfeeding is recommended, if possible, until nine, or at the latest, twelve months of age. For children with an increased risk of allergy — for example, owing to parents with allergies — it is even more important to breastfeed exclusively for the first six months, as this decreases the risk of allergic complaints. The gut matures progressively during the first year and can increasingly keep undigested substances out of the body. Children who are breastfed are rarely overweight. In addition, breastfeeding helps to establish a special bond between the mother and child.

Are there any disadvantages? One of the disadvantages that might be put forward is that it costs the mother a great deal of energy. She gives away a lot. Some mothers hardly notice this, but others feel exhausted after a few months; literally sucked dry.

Eating well and drinking a lot are important, but not the whole story. It is just as important to rest and take some time for yourself now and then. Admittedly, parents rarely manage to avoid losing out on sleep during the first few months, but you can make sure that this does not go too far by taking a nap in the afternoon, and perhaps asking people around you to help.

Taking time for yourself may seem more difficult, particularly when there are other children. However, if you can see how important this is, it is often possible to organize a few hours a week when you can do what you like. The practical aspects of breastfeeding are described in detail in the section with practical advice for different stages (see pp.55, 64, 72 and 80).

How long should you breastfeed?

Stopping breastfeeding can often be a difficult and emotional time. Mothers stop for different reasons. Sometimes, the child no longer seems interested in breastfeeding, for example, if she is given a lot of other food. In many cases, it is the mother who wants to stop because of her job, or because feeding is difficult, takes a great deal of energy, or simply because she thinks it is the right moment for her and for the child. Many mothers stop at an early stage, often because they have little help or support from the people around them. This is a pity, and continues to be a source of concern for baby clinics. Some mothers find feeding so easy and the baby enjoys it so much, that they seem able to go on forever, sometimes far beyond the first year. Looking at the child and her development, we feel that breastfeeding after the first year is no longer suitable for the particular stage the child is at, because the child is more independent. As regards the motor development of the mouth and the development of the teeth, it is important for a child to get used to eating from a spoon and swallowing from about five months, and later to start chewing thicker and coarser food. By nine months, children can often eat a sandwich; at this stage, sucking (either bottle-feeding or breastfeeding) is no longer appropriate for the newly acquired motor development of the mouth.

At the same time, the child is undergoing motor development, which means that from being completely dependent in the first few months, she becomes able to move independently, when she starts to crawl and walk. In this way, the child literally shows that she is separating herself from the mother, and we feel that stopping breastfeeding is suitable at this stage.

If you go on breastfeeding for longer than a year, the child becomes much more conscious of everything, including the breast producing the milk, which feels good to suck. In addition, a child of that age increasingly imposes her own will, and some children can start to insist very forcefully on being breastfed.

Bottle-feeding

If the baby is not breastfed, or if all the measures taken to stimulate breastfeeding are unsuccessful or inadequate (see p.60), the baby must be bottle fed. Giving a bowl of cereal to replace breastfeeding is not possible for the first few months, because it is too difficult to digest and the baby's sucking reflex is still too great.

There are many sorts of bottle-feeding; we will give a general summary here and list the advantages and disadvantages of the different types. Many changes are taking place in this field and it is always a good idea to discuss the matter at the baby clinic.

We make a distinction between using formula milk, and bottle feeds which you prepare yourself.

Formula milk, also known as *complete* baby food, is composed

in such a way that a baby does not need any solids up to the age of six months. Organic formula milks are now also available.

If you prepare the feed yourself, this makes use of diluted cow's milk with the addition of almond paste, lactose and eventually rice flour until six months of age and then wheat flour. If breastfeeding is entirely replaced by this type of bottle-feeding, it is necessary to start adding supplements in the form of fruit and vegetables at an early stage — that is, at about two months of age — in the form of two teaspoons of carrot (or other) juice daily.

Advantages and disadvantages
One advantage of formula milk is that it is a complete product which is generally well tolerated and easy to prepare.

One of the disadvantages is that it is an industrial product and is, therefore, not prepared with fresh ingredients. Furthermore, because of the many processes to which the basic raw materials are subjected, they are further removed from their natural origins than food that you prepare yourself. If parents prefer not to give their child vitamin K or vitamin D the disadvantage of this complete baby food is that these vitamins are added as standard.

In this book we are unable to discuss the various types of non-organic products for bottle-feeding in specific detail. There is a large range of 'ordinary' products on the market, as well as specific products for bottle-feeding children with feeding problems, which can be particularly useful for children with allergies to cow's milk or proteins, and should certainly be discussed at the baby clinic.

There is an important distinction between organic and non-organic formula milk. Organic formula products are based on organic cow's milk, which is a great advantage, particularly for babies, as it contains less pesticides. In addition to some vitamin K, less vitamin D is added to this product than to the non-organic bottle-feeding products. Thus there is still a choice to adapt the amount of vitamin D to the season to some extent, for example, only giving extra vitamin D during the winter months. Again, this should be discussed at the baby clinic.

The above-mentioned disadvantages of non-organic bottle-feeding with regard to processing also apply to organic feeding.

Since 1999, adding vitamin B1 has been compulsory in the EU for products sold as 'baby food.' As organic baby foods are generally richer in vitamin B1 than ordinary baby foods, and we believe that a varied, good quality diet contains enough vitamin B1, we do not support this EU regulation. The addition of vitamin B1 must be mentioned on the packaging. For some products, a temporary exception will apply. Look at the packaging to see whether or not vitamin B1 has been added.

'Next stage milk' (also called 'follow on' milk) is available for both organic and non-organic baby foods. This is recommended for children from the age of six months, because cow's milk, including diluted cow's milk, is allegedly too rich in minerals and too low in iron. In our opinion, healthy children are able to tolerate (diluted) cow's milk very well from six months, and a varied diet prepared using high quality ingredients will contain sufficient iron, even if the child eats a vegetarian diet.

For children with digestive problems, or children whose growth is slow, the next stage milk may be a good alternative.

It may be possible to find a formula milk made from goat's milk for children with digestive problems as well as children who are sensitive to cow's milk, as they are often able to tolerate this better.

One of the advantages of preparing bottles yourself, is that parents can prepare the bottle with products which have biodynamic or organic origins. In addition, vitamin K and vitamin D are not added as standard, so this also remains a choice you can make yourself. The preparation requires slightly more time than formula milk preparation.

One disadvantage is that it is necessary to start to supplement the diet with fruit and vegetables at a relatively young age. Preparing bottles yourself is not suitable for children who have difficulties with digestion, or who have an allergy problem.

Preparing bottles using almond paste as a base

The recipe for this bottle-feeding product aims to approximate the composition and nutritional value of mother's milk as closely as possible, taking into account the baby's digestive possibilities. For this purpose, cow's milk is greatly diluted for bottle-feeding babies up to the age of four months, and carbohydrates (in the form of lactose) and proteins and fats (in the form of almond paste) are added.

For babies over four months, the milk is not so diluted, and some rice flour (until 6 months) and cold-pressed sunflower or olive oil are added to the bottle. Boiled milk is less easily digested than unboiled pasteurised milk.

The milk is diluted as follows.

0–4 months	1 part full-fat milk to 2 parts water
4–6 months	1 part full-fat milk to 1 part water
6–8 months	2 parts full-fat milk to 1 part water
8 months +	undiluted

See Feeding Table, p 114

It was decided to add almonds to the product for bottle-feeding because they are easily digestible and can easily be mixed, as well as having a pleasant taste. Other nuts are less suitable in this respect. Furthermore, almonds are rich in fats, proteins and trace elements, which are a good supplement to the diluted milk used for bottle-feeding. Bottle-feeding using almond paste as a base originally came from Germany, where a university clinic found that it had positive results. Recipes for this type of bottle-feeding can be found in Chapters 3–6 at the end of each chapter.

We advise against using unpasteurised goat's milk rather than cow's milk to prepare the bottle-feeds because of the low folic acid content in goat's milk. Some brands add extra folic acid to their goat's milk.

Weaning

If the baby is breastfed, it is excellently fed and only really needs solids from about six months. Nevertheless, if allergies are not present, we advise starting to give solids slightly earlier. From four to five months the child becomes increasingly interested in the world about him and wants to explore this world. This need is met by providing fruit and vegetables. Being fed with a spoon is also a new experience.

For the child to learn to taste things, and for the digestive system to develop well, it is best to give

Root	Stem/leaves	Flower/fruit
carrot	cauliflower	broccoli
beetroot	spinach	pumpkin
Jerusalem artichoke	endive	courgette
parsnip	lamb's lettuce	peas
	salad greens	french beans
	leaf beet	runner beans
	fennel	mangetout
	kohlrabi	fruit
	pak choi	

each new type of fruit or vegetable for a few days in succession. When the child has become used to this, it is possible to try out a new fruit or vegetable. Then they can be alternated, or two vegetables can be combined. As far as possible, our preference is for fruit and vegetables which are in season, and which have been grown biodynamically or organically in the open ground. Greenhouse products should be used as little as possible.

Fruit and vegetables
When choosing vegetables it is a good idea to take into account the fact that plants consist of three elements — that is, the root system, the stem/leaves and the flower/fruit. A harmonious diet takes each of these three elements into account, either alternately or in combination with each other. In food crops one of the three elements is usually predominant. Fruit obviously represents the flower/fruit element. The practical section of this book indicates when a particular type of fruit or vegetable can be introduced.

Nitrates
Many vegetables — particularly green vegetables — naturally contain nitrates. As nitrates are partially converted in the body into *nitrites* and *nitrosamines,* which can be harmful to health, it is a good idea to take the nitrate content of different types of vegetables into account, particularly for very young babies.

Adults are much less at risk. The nitrate content of vegetables is influenced by the method of cultivation. The use of artificial fertilizers, as well as greenhouse cultivation out of season, increase the nitrate content. In general, organically and biodynamically grown vegetables contain fewer nitrates than conventionally grown vegetables. It is not

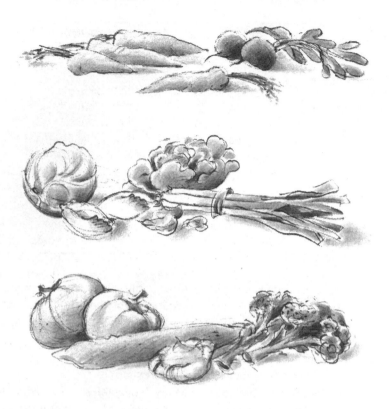

necessary to remove all vegetables containing nitrates from the diet. This would leave only a limited range of vegetables, and it is possible to keep the nitrate levels in the baby's diet low if a few general rules are observed:
— as far as possible, buy vegetables which are in season and which have been grown biodynamically or organically, and use only fresh products;
— do not give the baby any vegetables rich in nitrates before the age of six months;
— do not include vegetables rich in nitrates more than twice a week in the diet;

— cook vegetables rich in nitrates as quickly as possible (this does not apply for beetroot) and throw away the water they were cooked in. Never reheat the vegetables.

Vegetables low in nitrates are: cauliflower, broccoli, pumpkin, parsnip, Jerusalem artichoke, carrot, peas, french beans, runner beans, courgettes, mangetout.

Vegetables rich in nitrates are: endive (moderately rich in nitrates), lettuce, salad greens, leaf beet, beetroot, spinach, lamb's lettuce, fennel, kohlrabi.

Cereals

Cereals are the seeds of plants in which the three main elements are represented in a particularly harmonious way. Cereals have strong roots, a well-developed stem and powerful fruit/seeds, which ripen in the sun. This food crop can be combined with all the vegetables mentioned above.

Cereals can be added to the fruit or vegetables in the form of flakes or flour from the age of six to seven months. Up the age of six or seven months you should use cereals which do not contain gluten, because some children do not tolerate gluten very well. Cereals which are gluten-free include rice, maize and crops related to cereals, such as buckwheat and quinoa. Millet contains a substance similar to gluten, but this is usually tolerated very well.

After six or seven months it is possible to gradually introduce oats, barley and wheat; these cereals do contain gluten. Rye is only given after a few years.

Cereals are made digestible through a process of milling, rolling, soaking, cooking and simmering. Some of this is done in a factory, for example, milling or rolling the cereal to produce flakes, or processing cereals to make instant products. The rest in done at home in the kitchen. It is important to do this carefully because the small child's digestive system is still limited. Further instructions are given in Chapters 3–6.

Potatoes, pulses, meat and eggs

It is quite possible to ensure a good and balanced diet without potatoes, pulses, meat and eggs. Unlike true roots, potatoes are stem tubers that develop underground, in a kind of reversal of the principles governing a stem. Qualitatively, they have a different effect on the metabolism of a small child, and so we do not recommend them for babies.

Eggs, meat and to some extent, pulses, have a high protein content in contrast to breastmilk. This can accelerate physical growth and weight gain beyond what is appropriate for the slow maturation of human beings. For these reasons we do not recommend these foods for a small child's development.

A sweet tooth

Breast milk is naturally sweet, as it seems that a small child initially needs this sweet taste to be able to grow and thrive. Many parents prefer not to give their child anything sweet, even in a bottle, because they are afraid that the baby will get too used to the sweet taste. In fact, children who cannot do without sweets, sandwiches with sweet spreads, sweet puddings etc. share a common problem, which has a bad effect on their teeth and their health in general. However, the fear of getting used to sweet foods in the first year is not justified if the sweet taste is not overdone.

In the practical sections on feeding (see Chapters 3 and 4), only the almond bottle feeds and porridge are sweetened. All the foods can be given unsweetened. In the first few months, it is possible to use lactose, but later it is possible to choose between malt products (barley malt syrup, rice malt syrup) and maple syrup.

Salt and herbs

During the first year no salt should be added to the food. Salt, such as that which is found naturally in cow's milk, is sufficient; the baby would not be able to tolerate any more. Nor should any herbs from the garden be added to the food. The baby's voyage of discovery through the tastes of all the new foods is intensive enough in itself.

Heating up food

For the first year, all bottles and food are given at body temperature. *Vegetables* and *cereals* are always cooked. By *steaming* the vegetables rather than *boiling* them in water, the nutritional value is retained more effectively. Use a steamer or a metal colander placed on top of a pan with a small amount of boiling water, and a lid on top.

Raw vegetables are not given until after the baby is one year old. Cooking the food usually makes it easily digestible, but this does not apply to cow's milk, which should not be heated above body temperature in the first year, as it becomes too heavy

to digest. Pre-packaged milk, including organic milk, is pasteurised. The process of pasteurisation sterilizes the milk, which is a prerequisite for baby food, though it does not affect its digestibility.

Cooking *fruit* is not necessary, except at the very beginning. As it ripens, the fruit has already absorbed so much of the warmth of the sun that the baby will be able to digest uncooked fruit very easily.

Cook vegetables and cereals in a thick-bottomed pan so that the food cooks evenly, which will enhance its quality and taste.

It is not a good idea to heat food in a microwave or use food from the freezer. Both the microwave and the freezer remove vital qualities from the food, which a small baby needs. The microwave does not add warmth to the food, but shocks the stored warmth out of the product.

Puréeing the food

Solids should be puréed up to the age of eight to nine months. After that, it is possible to purée the food more coarsely, when bread is introduced. If the fruit or vegetable is suitable, it can be mashed.

A purée sieve (hand mincer) is best for preparing the food because it purées it, as well as removing parts of the food which are difficult for the child to digest. Electric hand mixers and food processors do not do this; they merely purée the food. This means that the fibres of some vegetables or cereals, which are difficult to digest, also end up in the baby food. They also beat air into the food, which can give some children wind or colic.

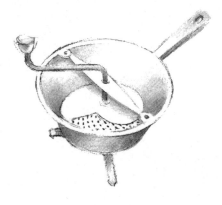

3. Practical Advice for Birth to Three Months

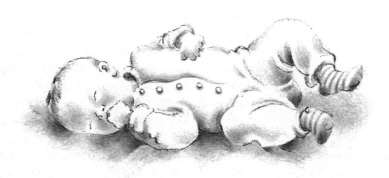

Psychomotor development

During the course of the first three months, the child gradually learns to control his head. In the first month he learns to focus, for example, on his father or mother. He also learns to follow an object, first with his eyes, and in the second month by rotating the head along with the eyes.

In the second month, the baby is able to hold up his head independently.

The baby starts to laugh at about six weeks, which is a real milestone for the baby and its parents.

In the second and third months, the baby learns to raise his chest as well as his head, when lying on his stomach.

Sleeping and waking

During the first three months, the baby is only really awake at the times that he is being fed. Adding up the time it takes to change the baby, this lasts from 45 minutes to up to one hour every time. By the end of these three months these periods may already be longer. If the baby's pattern of sleeping and waking is very different, for example, because he cries a lot and sleeps for short periods, or because he is difficult to wake, you should discuss this with the baby clinic.

Crying

Many babies cry quite regularly in the first three months. This is because they are getting used to a new life, and their intestines are still developing and usually cannot perform their functions straightaway. This can lead to hours of restlessness every day, as well as periods of crying. In general, restlessness or crying for two or three hours a day is quite normal. This does not mean to say that a restless or crying baby is easy to live with; it takes you over completely.

First of all, it is important to learn to distinguish different types of crying. If the baby grizzles while he is falling asleep, this can be ignored for a while because it often stops automatically. If the baby is crying because he is cross and cannot settle, this also often stops after a while. Sometimes the baby will turn red. There are many children who fall asleep this way. However, there are some babies who cry so much that you simply have to console them because they cannot settle on their own.

Over the course of the first three weeks, the parent will start to hear whether the baby is crying because he has wind, or is troubled by a dirty nappy (diaper), or because he is hungry. Obviously something has to be done about this.

The most common cause of crying mentioned by parents is cramp. You cannot always tell from the baby's position — curled up with his legs tucked up — because all babies lie like this when they cry a lot. The way in which he cries — vehemently, often alternating with short periods of silence — can tell you more, particularly if the crying is accompanied by a hard and swollen stomach and a lot of wind. At the baby clinic you can discuss whether to make any changes if you are breastfeeding. If the baby is bottle fed it is best not to change to a different sort of formula milk straightaway if the baby has cramp; changes in feeding can exacerbate cramps. There are a number of ways that can help with crying babies. Again it is important not to try everything out on one day, but to try out one thing for a few days to see whether it helps.

The method of feeding

In the case of breastfeeding, problems can arise if the baby has developed the wrong technique for drinking; for example, if the baby drinks too greedily and messily, so that he sucks in air. It often helps to hold the baby in a more vertical position. If the baby drinks too greedily, it can be helpful to express some milk before feeding. The baby can then drink more calmly.

If the baby is fed too often once breastfeeding has started, and does not empty either of the breasts fully, he may be getting too much fore milk. This is rich in carbohydrate, in contrast with the hind milk, which contains more fat. If the baby is proportionally drinking more fore milk than hind milk, this can lead to fermentation in the intestines.

In the case of bottle-feeding, the hole in the teat may be too large, so that the baby gets a lot of food in a short time. Look at the quantity: is the baby getting too much or too little (see Feeding Table on p.114). Swaddling is an effective procedure for restless and crying babies (see also p.108)

It also makes a big difference if you are able to deal with crying in a fairly relaxed way. If you are able to communicate a feeling of calm and tranquillity and establish a pattern in your behaviour, this will also calm down the child.

Page 99 describes a number of household remedies, which may help for stomach cramps.

If you are worried about the crying and think that something is really wrong with the baby, contact your doctor or the baby clinic.

Care

Bathing and washing

Bathing the baby daily is not really necessary and is actually inadvisable in the first few weeks after birth. Once or twice a week is usually sufficient. In fact, the baby loses a great deal of warmth when bathed, and not all babies feel comfortable when they are completely undressed to have a bath. Furthermore, the layer of sebum, which is of enormous importance to the baby for the first few days after birth because it feeds and protects the skin, will soak off when the baby is bathed. If you do not bath the baby, you should obviously give him a wash every day instead.

Bathing
Bathing the baby safely and efficiently is quite an art, which is usually learnt with the help of a health professional just after the baby is born. It is important for the room in which the baby is bathed to be well heated, and to wrap the clean clothes and towel around a hot water bottle beforehand. An extra hot water bottle should also be placed in the cot so that the bedding remains warm. This should be removed before the baby is placed in the cot.

Do not leave the baby in the bath too long. Pat the baby dry all over and dress him quickly. As bathing is tiring, the baby will often fall asleep straightaway after he has had a bath and been fed.

Washing
When you wash the baby, do not undress him completely, but undress him bit by bit to prevent him

from cooling down. Only those parts of the body that really need it are washed; the rest can be cleaned when the baby is bathed. Wash the face, ears, folds of the neck, armpits and diaper (nappy) area carefully with water, pat dry and apply calendula baby oil or another hypoallergenic product, as it provides a protective film on the skin. Do not clean inside the ears.

There is no need to use soap, because it removes too much oil from the skin. The diaper area, armpits and folds of the neck can also be cleaned with some cotton wool and baby oil (see above). Ready-to-use baby wipes sometimes cause irritation to the baby's bottom.

Nails

In the first few weeks it is only necessary to cut the baby's nails if he scratches himself. Cut the nails straight and not too short with a special pair of baby scissors or baby nail clippers. Do this at a moment when the baby is quiet or asleep.

Foreskin

In little boys, the foreskin does not usually move freely yet. Nothing has to be done about this; until the age of six, simply wash and pat dry.

Umbilical cord

In general, the umbilical cord drops off between the fourth and fourteenth day. By six weeks, the navel is usually dry. In principle, you do not have to do anything apart from keeping the navel as dry and clean as possible. In order to help it dry up, it is possible to use some Weleda Wecesin powder in the navel several times a day. Continue to use this, even after the umbilical cord has dropped off, until the skin of the navel is dry and looks clean. Make sure that the baby does not breathe in the powder when you are applying it.

Taking the baby's temperature

During the first few days after the birth, take the baby's temperature every day. The temperature should be about 37°C (98.6°F). Taking the baby's temperature during the first few days is important because it takes a while for the baby to start to regulate his own body temperature, and one blanket or one hot water bottle (not in the cot with the child) more or less will have an immediate influence on its temperature.

After this, you should get to know the baby so well that it is only necessary to take his temperature when he is ill (see p.24f). Observing the baby closely is important, because each child is different, and because the weather can change the baby's temperature very rapidly.

If the baby really feels the cold, an extra bonnet, even in the cradle, sometimes works better than an extra blanket, because much warmth can be lost from the baby's relatively large head.

Diapers (nappies)

For parents who like to use cotton nappies (because cotton is good for the skin, or for the sake of the environment), but cannot cope with the mountains of washing, there are nappy services available. These organizations collect the dirty cotton nappies from your home and bring clean ones in their place.

Wrap the baby up in a woollen wrap over the cotton nappy, or put knitted woollen overpants over the cotton nappy. These keep the baby warm and let very little moisture through, although they do breathe.

In the cot

During the first two weeks, it is important to put the baby alternately on one side, then on the other side, then on his back. The effects of gravity, to which the baby is now exposed for the first time, can affect the shape of his head, as well as the relationship between his trunk and pelvis. By changing the baby's position, you can avoid too much pressure on one side.

Since the first results were published in the Netherlands in 1989 about the link between placing babies on their stomach and cot death, all baby clinics advise against this position. Infant mortality rates have clearly fallen as a result. After the age of two to three weeks, it is not advisable to place a baby on his side, because he can then roll onto his stomach. It is therefore advisable to place him on his back at this stage. Since this advice has been given, there have been an increasing number of babies with flattened heads. This does not do any damage to the brain. As regards the appearance: as soon as the baby starts to play lying on his stomach in the playpen and starts to sit up, the shape of the skull will change back to some extent. Any flatness that remains will not be so noticeable once the hair grows.

Some children develop a preference for lying on their back with their head to one side. This can result in the back of the head not only becoming flat, but also slightly crooked. It is possible to take a number of measures to prevent this. Turn the cot around; the changing light and the new direction from which adults approach the cot can sometimes have a corrective influence. When you change the baby, place him directly in front of you instead of at an angle to emphasize symmetry. These measures may not always be successful. Discuss the problem with the doctor if you are worried.

As a preventative measure to safeguard against cot death, it is advisable for the baby to sleep in his own cot, not in his parents' bed. Many parents like the baby to sleep in their room, especially for the first few weeks or months. This feels safe and is easy if the baby is still having night feeds. The time at which the baby moves into his own room (if there is one) to sleep will depend on the parents' needs and on the baby's sleeping pattern (also see Night feeds, p.56). During the day, the baby should be allowed to sleep in a quiet room. It does not have to be absolutely silent, because children generally sleep well in a room where household sounds can penetrate to some extent. However, it should be somewhere where the baby can be quiet, without being constantly stimulated, thus preventing it from sleeping. Therefore, a bedroom is much more suitable for sleeping than the living room, particularly for babies who are awake a lot or easily stimulated. At first it may seem that the baby is rather a long way away, but experience has shown that you can still feel the connection with your baby at a distance.

Many parents use a baby monitor at home to feel secure. The disadvantage of this is that you respond to every sound the child makes. Babies make all sorts of sounds while they are asleep, and these may seem rather alarming through a baby monitor. This means that many parents take the baby out of the cot to calm him down, but this can actually make him restless and stop him from learning to solve minor problems for himself.

The room where the baby sleeps should be thoroughly aired at least once a day. Apart from this, the temperature of the room should be between 18°C and 20°C (64°–68°F). If the baby is able to keep himself warm and is growing well, the temperature of the room can drop to about 15°C (60°F). During this stage, it is often necessary to pre-warm the cot with hot water bottles.

Going outside

For the first few weeks after the birth, there is no need for the baby to go outside. When he laughs for the first time, it shows that he is starting to feel at home here on earth. This may be the moment at which the baby can gradually get used to going outside. A baby does not need direct sunlight, not even to prevent rickets (see p.84). Too much sunlight on the skin can be dangerous, leading to sunburn and dehydration in the short term, and permanent damage to the skin in the long term.

The best place when the baby is outside in the pram in the shade under a blue sky; but if it is overcast, a baby can still come into contact with light and air. Light and air are essential for the baby's development; first, held in his parent's arms, and then in the pram in good weather. If you have a garden, the baby can sleep outside in the pram. In summer it is important to ensure that the baby does not become overheated under the hood of the pram. If this is the case, place the pram in the shade. Take the way in which the wind is blowing into account. In general, children sleep very well outside.

Always stay nearby, because warm prams are very attractive to cats, and use a cat net.

If you take the baby outside in winter, it is important to dress him warmly.

Thumb sucking and dummies

Between the age of six weeks and three months, many babies discover their thumb and start sucking it. When the baby sucks his thumb, this helps him to make contact with himself, and withdraw into a dreamy inner world. Thumb sucking can be a consolation and have a calming influence.

In the first few weeks, babies often cry, sometimes a great deal, because entering a new life is by no means easy. A thumb could be a great consolation but the baby has to find his thumb himself, and this often takes a long time.

A dummy can serve as an alternative to the thumb. We would like to briefly outline the advantages and disadvantages.

Thumb sucking

A child always has his thumb with him, and can put it in his mouth when he feels the need to do so. Dentists have different views about the negative effects which frequent thumb sucking could have on the jaw. A child has to learn to stop sucking his thumb by himself, preferably before the permanent teeth come through, and this can be quite difficult.

If thumb sucking is linked with a cuddly toy or doll, it could be limited by only having the toy in the cot.

Dummies

The great disadvantage of dummies is that the child is dependent on his parents. If the baby loses the dummy in the cot, he will not be able to find it by himself. Crying is the only way of letting the parents know, and this may happen several times a night. If the baby uses the dummy a lot when he is not in the cot, this can affect the healthy motor development of the mouth and speech. Do not give the baby a dummy if he has not become used to the breast and has not really mastered the sucking technique. By sucking on the dummy in this situation, the baby can learn the wrong sucking technique. If you give the baby a dummy, the flat, broad variety is preferable to the round, cherry-shaped model in connection with the development of the jaw. It should definitely be removed when children start to speak as they might develop a lisp.

Hiccups

There can be different causes for the hiccups. Too much food all at once, or food that is too cold can cause hiccups, but so can stress or too much excitement. Copper ointment can be a good remedy if the hiccups lead to a great deal of restlessness. Apply some copper ointment to the stomach with a warm hand, and at the same height on the back.

Toys and playing

The child learns to explore the world through direct sensory contact — with his ears, nose, mouth, eyes, skin and hands, he assimilates everything. During these months these are his toys. For example, the baby will discover his own hands and will practise endlessly bringing them together.

The parent's face is also fascinating to look at or touch; the nose, hair, and mouth. If you make sounds, recite a nursery rhyme or sing softly, the child will watch and listen intently.

When the baby is outside in the pram he can look at the rustling leaves in the tree. He will see shadows and light and feel warm or cool air on his skin. His pleasure can be further increased by an attractive ribbon on the branch of a tree or shrub, or a bell to play with.

Safety

The most common accidents during this period are caused by burns, falls and suffocation. Take the following precautions:

Burns

Always check the hot water bottle and make sure that is it never in direct contact with the baby. It is best to place the hot water bottle between two blankets at the foot of the cot, and remove before placing the baby in the cot.

Make sure that the bath water is at body temperature.

Falls

Never leave the baby alone, even for just a moment on the dressing table, or on a bed without a rail.

Use a changing mat with a raised edge on the dressing table.

When you walk around holding the baby, make sure that there are no articles left lying around on the floor or the stairs that you may trip over.

Suffocation or strangling

Make sure that there are no small objects left around the baby, such as loose drawstrings on clothes or hats, or, for example, electric cable near the cot; any drawstrings on the clothes should be well secured.

When you use a bonnet, check that the bonnet encloses the head properly, and the cord is securely fastened. It is better to tie it firmly with a short drawstring than to have a loose knot.

Also make sure that the lining of the cot is properly secured, and do not use a duvet.

In the first few years, it is not advisable to use a pillow in the cot, from the point of view of safety.

Feeding

Breastfeeding

Breastfeeding is the art of giving, an art which you learn particularly in the first few weeks. In order to be able to give, the mother must be relaxed, or the reflex which releases the milk from the supply behind the nipple will not occur satisfactorily.

A quiet environment contributes to a relaxed feeling, both for yourself and for the baby. Try to feed the baby in the room where he sleeps as much as possible, particularly in the beginning, without household noises around you and without any visitors. A relaxed position is also very important when you are feeding the baby.

The position for feeding

Lying down: Place your shoulder on the mattress and your head on the pillow. Draw up your upper leg and support your knee with the mattress. Make sure that you both feel comfortably warm, and if necessary take another blanket or duvet.

Sitting down: Place a pillow on your lap or under your arm for the baby to lie on so that you do not have to carry him in your arms all the time; a foot rest means that you do not have to cross your legs to keep the baby at the right height. Make sure that when you are feeding the baby, his head and body are in a straight line or that his stomach is lying against you. If his head is turned away from the body, it is much more difficult to swallow.

The rhythm of feeding

Breastfeeding is a matter of supply and demand. The more often you feed the baby, the more milk will be produced. It usually takes a few weeks before supply and demand are interrelated. Insisting on a rhythm too rigidly during this period, with not enough times when the baby can feed, could prevent the pattern for breastfeeding from developing satisfactorily. The baby's own feeding rhythm starts to emerge after the first few weeks. This is often approximately every three or four hours, but hardly ever at exact intervals. For example, a pattern may emerge with three and a half or four hours between every feed in the morning, and three hours in the afternoon. This is the baby's own rhythm. If there is a clear pattern, use this as a starting point for the next few weeks and try to keep to the routine as far as possible.

A good routine creates a peaceful, calm atmosphere; parents often say that their children flourish better with a clear routine than with feeding on demand. This rhythm may be as follows: five to six times during the day, that is, every three or four hours, and another feed during the night if the baby wakes up for it.

One or two breasts

As indicated above, breastfeeding is a matter of supply and demand. The more often you breastfeed the baby, the better lactation is stimulated. In principle, it is therefore advisable for the baby to drink from both breasts during every feed. It is important that at least one of the breasts is completely emptied so that the baby gets some of the more fatty milk which is produced after the colostrum and is more nourishing. If the baby appears to be hungry fairly soon after the previous feed, start with the emptiest breast, and then go back to the full breast as the first one at the normal feeding time.

Night feeds

The baby often develops an awareness of night and day for the first time at about six weeks, and the gap between the night feeds can be gradually increased.

Parents can work towards this by feeding the baby briefly and in a 'businesslike manner' at night, and by keeping the light and sound low, that is, by feeding in a very different atmosphere from the daytime. When the baby shows that it can sleep for five or six hours at a time, but still wakes up too early, for example, at 5 o'clock instead of 7 o'clock, there are several ways to help it take the last step in the right direction:

— only change the baby's nappy and then place him back in the cot;

— give a bottle with approximately 100 ml (3½ fl oz) of fennel or camomile tea (see the recipes on p.110). The baby is satisfied because he has had something, but will wake up for the next feed within two hours, so that his routine is maintained.

— move the cot from the parents' bedroom to another room; very often, parents who have become used to night feeds will prevent the baby from sleeping because they are tossing and turning.

It is certainly advisable to give the first morning feed at a set time, or to work towards this, even if the night feed changes, for example, from 3 o'clock in the morning to 5 o'clock in the morning. In this way, a routine is maintained.

Crying with hunger

As you get to know your baby, you will also start to recognise why he is crying (see also p.48). Crying with hunger is one reason to forget about the pattern of feeding and to feed the baby more often, particularly when this happens several times. Usually, by feeding the baby quite often it takes one or two days to establish a new pattern, which will be enough for the amount of milk to adapt to the baby's needs. Then it is possible to return to the first feeding pattern.

Bowel movements

A baby's stools are black and sticky for the first few days (meconium). Then the stools of breastfed babies usually acquire a creamy yellow, sometimes green consistency. A baby may have from seven dirty nappies a day to just one a week. Different colours and amounts can also be quite normal. There may also be quite a difference in the thickness of the stools, but in babies who are breastfed they are usually thinner, and never really very thick. It is quite normal for a baby to be completely covered with excrement when it has pushed hard for a while. It can only really be characterised as diarrhea when it is very watery with just a few solid bits, and occurs more than six times a day. If a baby only moves its bowels once or a few times a week, it may become a problem and have a negative influence on the drinking pattern, while the stools that are produced are rarely very thick. In this case, mildly laxative foods may help. The mother could eat some dried prunes, or drink some orange juice. If this does not help, or if the orange juice causes cramps or gives the baby a red bottom, give the baby some of the water in which the prunes were soaked, and discuss the problem at the baby clinic.

Weighing the baby

In the UK, it is recommended that babies are weighed at birth, at two weeks and at six weeks. The birth weight should be regained within two or at most three weeks. If a good feeding pattern is established in the following period, the baby should have at least six very wet nappies per day, and if he is happy, then it is no longer necessary to weigh him at home. If you use disposable nappies it is difficult to assess how wet they are — particularly when you have your first child. If you have any doubts about whether the amount of food that the baby is receiving is sufficient, don't look only at whether or not the baby is happy but also use the scales. There are babies who remain quiet even if they are hungry. Therefore we advise weighing the baby naked twice a week until the first visit to the baby clinic.

Yellow skin

Many babies have a slightly yellow colour in the first few days after they are born because of the increased bilirubin content of the body. This usually disappears without any problems within a few days. If the baby is very yellow and seems sleepy and difficult to wake up, it is important to make sure he comes into contact with daylight, for example, by placing the cot by a (closed) window with the hood back. In addition, it is important for the child to drink a lot. Feed him at least eight times a day, even when this may be difficult because the baby is sleepy. It is not advisable to supplement the feed with water, tea or glucose water. Breastfeeding, particularly the first feed, has a laxative effect, so that the meconium containing the bilirubin is soon removed from the intestines.

The mother's diet

Altogether drink approximately one litre more per day than you usually do; for example, herbal teas, fruit juice, milk and milk products and tea which stimulates lactation. Approximately 500ml (half quart) of dairy products per day is sufficient.

If possible, eat foods which have not been sprayed, and have been thoroughly cooked; for example, easily digestible cereals, bread, sufficient dairy products, cheese or meat, nuts (almonds). For the first six weeks, avoid vegetables which cause wind or are difficult to digest (brassicas and leeks), spicy meals and citrus fruits. After this, you can gradually see whether the baby will tolerate these foods indirectly through the mother's milk. If the baby suffers from cramp, wind or posseting, it is also possible to see whether coarse, indigestible muesli, wholemeal bread or rye bread, which are difficult to digest, or raw vegetables and whole grains of wheat, rye or barley, should be removed from the diet for a while.

Avoid alcohol and nicotine (inhibits breastfeeding), as well as icy and/or carbonated drinks. Do not drink a lot of coffee or black tea. Always consult the doctor if you are taking medication.

Some practical tips

— If you have the impression that the baby does not have a good sucking technique or is too tired to drink, ask your midwife or health visitor for advice. For these questions, members of the National Childbirth Trust or the La Leche League, or a lactation expert, can give good advice; see the Useful Organizations on p.119.

— If you would like to give the baby his last feed just before you go to bed yourself, and it is difficult to wake him up, try to feed him while he is still asleep. Some babies can drink while they are asleep.

— Only use water to wash your nipples, not soap.

— Make sure that you are dressed warmly and that your arms are covered, when you are feeding. This helps to prevent mastitis.

— If you are troubled by constipation, there is usually no objection to eating some soaked dried prunes. If this does not help, and you are really drinking enough (2 litres / quarts or more per day), ask the doctor for advice.

— During the time that you are breastfeeding, try not to lose too much weight. All the harmful substances that we ingest with our food are stored in the form of fat. If a lot of fat is broken down — because you are slimming — these substances will find their way directly into the milk.

— If you plan to go back to work, it is best to discuss this at the baby clinic in good time, so you can ask for advice, for example, about expressing milk. It is quite an art to learn how to do this. In addition, the baby will have to learn to accept a bottle. From six weeks, give him a bottle of expressed milk once every one or two days, so that the baby is really used to the bottle by the time you start work.

Problems with breastfeeding

Cracked nipples

Cracked nipples are usually the result of breastfeeding incorrectly, or a poor sucking technique as a result of thrush, and sometimes as a result of the mother's sensitive skin. Thrush in particular is an increasingly common cause, which is not always recognised (see 'white spots' p.99). Ask your health professional for help in good time, rather than endlessly trying to solve the matter yourself with nipple pads etc.

It is a good idea to feed the baby often and for short periods. Whatever you do, do not postpone feeding the baby because it hurts; in fact, a baby does not suck so hard if the breast is less full.

After feeding the baby, rub the last drops of milk over the nipples with clean hands, as this can have a healing effect (do not do this if the baby has thrush). Make sure that the nipples are thoroughly dry, possibly by drying them with a hair dryer, and if necessary, wear a small metal sieve (without a handle) in your bra so that air can get to the nipples.

In addition, there is a whole series of ointments and tinctures such as Weleda calendula ointment, or mecurialis ointment or tincture. The advantage of tinctures is that the nipples do not become soft and the air can get to them. An ointment can be helpful for dry nipples, provided it is applied thinly after feeding the baby. Discuss this with your health professional.

Mastitis

If you suffer flu-like symptoms, have a fever and feeding the baby hurts, you are probably suffering from incipient mastitis. You can get mastitis if you are extremely tired, in combination with catching cold, as a result of cracked nipples, if the breast is not properly emptied, and also when you reduce the number of feeds, for example, when the night feed comes to an end.

It is never possible to completely empty the breast — you can always express some more milk — but it is not good if dried milk remains on the nipples after the feed. You must certainly go on feeding following the same pattern as before, or even slightly more often. If possible, start with the painful breast. However, if this is really too painful or if the milk does not come through, start with the healthy breast until the milk comes through, and then change to the painful breast.

Other remedies are:
— Before feeding, direct a hot shower at the breast or place something hot on it while you are feeding, so that milk flows more easily.
—After every feed place a compress

of curds on the painful spot for about thirty minutes. To do this, spread some curds at room temperature on a piece of muslin or thin handkerchief, and fold over the material.

— Instead of using a curd compress, you can also place some slightly bruised cabbage leaves (green or white cabbage) on the painful spot. Leave the leaves in position for a number of hours by placing them inside your bra.

— Ring the doctor if your fever has not gone down after one day. Mastitis can be easily treated with anthroposophical medicines without influencing milk production and without any harmful effects for the baby.

Too little milk

If the breasts do not feel really full, or if they produce a rather glassy, bluish milk rather than white milk, this does not mean that breastfeeding is inadequate. The composition of the milk changes over the months, and in principle, the quality is always good. After a while, the pressure in the breasts disappears once a good balance has been achieved between supply and demand. If the quantity of milk is not enough, you will see this more accurately from the baby's crying, the number of wet nappies per day and/or the baby's increase in weight. (See also p.57 under Weighing the baby).

The causes of not having enough milk can be incorrect breastfeeding or sucking technique, stress in the mother, too much restlessness when feeding, not giving enough feeds, giving only one breast every feed, the mother not drinking enough and overtiredness.

What can be done? Feed the baby more often, always give him both breasts. Make sure you rest enough yourself, and also eat enough. Do not start bottle-feeding too quickly, because the more often and the more powerfully the baby sucks, the better the breastfeeding will be.

Remedies which help the milk to flow include special teas, or Weleda's *Species lactagogae* (tea), oil to rub on the breasts (available on prescription from the doctor), sloe juice or elixir and almonds. Avoid parsley, sage and lemons as they reduce the flow of milk.

In some cases, none of this will help, for example, in a busy family with lots of children. In this case, accepting the fact and introducing bottle-feeding will relax everyone.

Too much milk

If there is always pressure on the breasts there is a danger of mastitis, or if the baby cannot cope with the supply of milk, drink slightly less and try to change to giving one breast every feed. If there is a lot of pressure, use cabbage leaves in the way described for mastitis. If this does not help, ask the nurse for advice.

Bottle-feeding

The advice given below applies for babies who are completely bottle fed. If you breastfeed as well as giving the bottle, you can see how much milk the baby is drinking from the breast, for example, by weighing the baby once a week, before and after a number of feeds. Adapt the amount given in the bottle accordingly.

Amount

During the first three months, the average requirement per day is 150 to 175 ml per kg of body weight (about $2^1/2$ oz per lb). In other words, for a baby weighing 4 kg, this amounts to 600 to 700 ml per day (20–24 fl oz). Obviously this quantity is gradually built up, starting on the first day after birth with six to seven times 10 to 15 ml (2–3 tsp), then six to seven times 20 to 30 ml (4–6 tsp) on the second day, and so on.

If you make use of formula milk, follow the instructions on the packaging.

A recipe for bottle-feeding based on almond paste and cow's milk is given below (see box below). If you change from formula milk to bottles you have prepared yourself, this must be done gradually, for example, by replacing one bottle per day.

Bottle-feeding based on almond paste for 0–3 months

Ingredients for 100 ml (or for 8 fl oz) bottle-feeding:
2 parts water, (65–70 ml, 5–$5^1/2$ fl oz)
1 part full-fat cow's milk (30–35 ml, $2^1/2$–3 fl oz)
4 g (2 tsp) white almond paste
6 g (1 tbsp) lactose

Boil the water. Remove the pan from the hob. Whisk the almond paste and lactose into the water so that the ingredients are thoroughly dissolved. Stir in the milk and pour everything through a tea strainer so that the bottle teat will not be obstructed by any lumps.

The full amount for the day can be prepared at the same time. Immediately after preparing the bottles, cool them down under cold running water and keep them carefully sealed in the fridge. Before feeding the baby, bring the desired quantity up to body temperature by heating the bottle in a pan of hot water or in a bottle warmer.

NB: This bottle-feeding is only adequate if fruit and vegetables are given from two months of age.

TIP: It is useful to weigh a spoonful of lactose or almond paste once, so that you can then use that particular spoon to measure the quantities in future.

The recipe for this type of bottle-feeding does not change for the next three months, although the quantity has to be adapted regularly (see Feeding Table, p.114). From about six weeks the night feed can be dropped, and five feeds should be sufficient.

Hygiene

For the first six months, it is particularly important to ensure hygiene as carefully as possible when cleaning the bottles and preparing the bottle feeds.

Immediately after use, rinse out the bottles with water. Boil the bottles once every two to three days in boiling water for ten minutes. Also rinse the teat after every feed with hot water, and boil them every two or three days for three minutes. Always keep the teats in a sealed jam jar. Replace the bottle teats every six weeks.

Bowel movements

In principle, a baby who is bottle fed should move his bowels every day, in contrast with a child who is breastfed. If he does not move his bowels as often as this, real problems can arise with constipation (see also p.101) Discuss this at the baby clinic in good time so that feeding can be adapted.

Solids with bottle-feeding

If the baby is not breastfed at all, but is fed with bottles prepared with almond paste, start with carrot juice, possibly mixed with apple juice, at about two months of age. Fresh juice is easy to make yourself, by grating a carrot or apple very finely and expressing the juice with the rounded side of a spoon. You can also use a piece of muslin or clean handkerchief and place the grated carrot or apple on this. Make it into a little bag and press out the juice.

Start with a few teaspoons, possibly diluted with water, and give this before the second or third bottle. At a later stage, this can be increased to a maximum of two dessertspoonfuls per day. Depending on the season, it is then possible to add juice made from blackcurrants, rose hips or tangerines. The juice of blueberries has a constipating effect.

Always makes sure that the solids are at body temperature.

Vaccinations

Discuss the subject of inoculations during one of your first visits to the baby clinic so that you have time to form an opinion (see also p.87ff).

3. Practical Advice for Three to Six Months

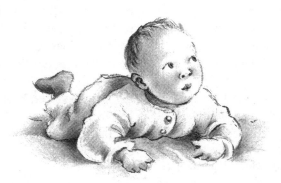

Psychomotor development

During this stage, learning to use the arms, hands and trunk are a priority.

From about four months the baby learns to use her hands, lying on her back — first just one hand, and then both hands at the same time. The child learns to move objects from one hand to the other. She will put everything she takes hold of into her mouth and explore it with great joy. The child learns that every object feels or tastes different, that there are different shapes, sizes and weights, and that some toys are warm while others are cold.

At about six months the child learns to raise herself up to her navel when she is lying on her stomach. The head is stable, and in this position she can look around at the world until she accidentally rolls over.

Supported by her father's or mother's arm, the child can sit up briefly, but is still much too small to be put in a baby chair or any other type of chair. During this stage, she learns to respond to the environment in a clear and focused way, and demonstrates this contact by gurgling contentedly.

Sleeping and waking

A day and night routine has usually been established by now, as the night feed stops. By the end of these months when the late feed has also been dropped, the baby will sleep through the night.

The rest of the sleeping and waking routine is still entirely related to the pattern of feeding. The baby will always sleep for two or three hours between feeds. The night starts after the 7 o'clock feed in the evening, and may be briefly interrupted for the late feed, as long as this remains necessary.

Care

The playpen

From four months it advisable to place the playpen in the living room. A playpen is a safe environment with firm boundaries for the child, and they can be contained with in their own area. Experiencing a boundary works psychologically by creating a shelter, which influences physical development in a positive way (See also p.31).

Dribbling

From the age of three months, many babies start to dribble, and by five months may dribble a lot. This dribbling does not always indicate that they are teething, but is usually a sign of developing salivary glands. A bib will keep the baby's top dry and prevent the child from cooling down.

Toys and playing

Now that the baby can hold something in her hand, a rattle, a knitted woollen ball with a bell inside her, or a cuddly toy are suitable toys.

The cuddly toy does not have to be any more than a square piece of cloth tied together. The baby explores everything with her mouth to find out about the world, bit by bit. In this way, she learns where her own body ends and the world begins.

'Itsy bitsy spider' is a favourite finger game.

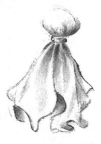

Safety

The most common accidents during this period are the same as those during the period between birth and three months (see p.54).

However, we would like to mention a few further points for attention: during this period, the baby learns to take hold of things, and it is therefore even more important to be careful with loose covers over the cot, pieces of cord and small objects in the cot, on the dressing table or in the playpen. The playpen must be safe. Take care to check the hinges.

Feeding

The pattern of feeding

In most cases, a clear feeding pattern has become established by the age of three months. The usual feeding times are 7 and 11 o' clock in the morning, 3 o' clock in the afternoon, and 7 and 11 o' clock in the evening. By the end of this stage, the 11 o'clock feed in the evening is usually dropped.

Breastfeeding

By the age of three months, the baby may no longer breastfeed quite as well. This is related to her growing interest in everything around her. It is typical for the baby to drink for a little bit, and then look at the mother with the breast still half in her mouth, laughing radiantly, then taking another sip, laughing again, and so on.

It helps if the mother does not give up and does not become irritated or angry. If possible, feed the baby in a quiet place with as few distractions as possible, and while the baby is feeding, do not respond to her beaming attempts to make contact.

Weaning

In the UK, health visitors advise that solids are given from six months if possible, and that babies are breastfed on demand.

To teach a baby to learn to eat from a spoon, it is useful to start with a small flat spoon, and to offer it only when the baby opens her mouth. Place the spoon horizontally in the mouth and then remove it horizontally without emptying it against the upper lip. This means that the baby will be more inclined to empty the spoon herself and swallow, rather than slurping and sucking. In the beginning she may well choke on the food a little. As the food is in a soft puréed form, there is no danger of really choking. After coughing a bit, most babies will be prepared to take further spoonfuls.

As soon as you start giving solids, the colour and smell of the stools will change. Vegetables will particularly change the colour.

Start with *fruit:* Raw, puréed apple or pear, and then add some juice from a sweet orange, a little bit of banana, or depending on the season, some blackcurrant or blueberry juice. If the baby finds it difficult to digest, start with cooked apple for the first two weeks. If this does not lead to any problems with breastfeeding, the food can be given before the third or fourth feed. However, if the baby no longer wants to drink from the breast or drinks significantly less after this supplement, give the food after breastfeeding.

Gradually increase the quantity from two teaspoonfuls to two dessertspoonfuls.

From five to six months, you can start giving some *vegetables* as well as fruit. In this case, give the fruit before (or if necessary, after) the third feed and the vegetables before (or if necessary, after) the second feed. Start with carrots.

Gradually increase the quantity from two teaspoonfuls to two dessertspoonfuls.

Once the baby has got used to carrots, you can also gradually introduce *cauliflower, broccoli and pumpkin,* either combined with the familiar carrots, or on their own.

A taste of fruit

Raw puréed apple: peel the apple and grate it finely with a nutmeg grater. If you use an ordinary grater this usually produces slivers rather than smooth purée.

Boiled apple purée: cook the peeled, finely diced apple in a little bit of water and purée the apple with the cooking liquid.
A taste of vegetables

Boil or steam (see p.44) pieces of vegetable in a little bit of water until they are thoroughly cooked and pass them through a sieve. If necessary, make the purée slightly thinner with some boiled water.

Bottle-feeding

Feeding schedule
7am—bottle of 170–200 ml (6–7 fl oz)
11am—vegetables + bottle of approx. 170 ml (6 fl oz)
3pm—fruit + bottle of approx. 170 ml (6 fl oz)
7pm—bottle of 170–200 ml (6–7 fl oz)
11pm—bottle of 170–200 ml (6–7 fl oz)

These times serve as a guideline and will differ from child to child.

In general, the last feed can be dropped between the ages of five and six months. This feed is then divided over the four bottles which the child has during the daytime.

If a child receiving formula milk indicates that she is no longer satisfied by the bottle during the course of this period, you can add some rice flour to the bottle. This can be the flour used for bottles which you prepare yourself.

For bottle-feeding with bottles you prepare yourself, you can use the recipe, *Bottle-feeding based on almond paste* (see p.61), up to four months.

From four months, add flour to this bottle so that the baby will be satisfied. This recipe is shown opposite.

Weaning with bottle-feeding

Up to three months, bottle-fed babies are given only carrot juice or fruit juice as supplements. Now it is possible to go on to puréed vegetables and fruit. For this, see the advice given under *Solids with breastfeeding* (see p.65) For a child who is bottle fed it is possible to deduct one month from the indicated age, because weaning started at a much earlier stage.

Bottle-feeding based on almond paste for 4–6 months

Ingredients per 100 ml (per 8 fl oz):
50 ml (4 fl oz) full-fat cow's milk
50 ml (4 fl oz) water
2 g (1 tsp) rice flour
4 g (2 tsp) lactose
3 g (1½ tsp) almond paste

Preparation with rice flour:
Cook the flour in the water until it is cooked (see instructions on the packaging) and dilute the lactose and almond paste in the warm liquid. Stir in the milk and pour everything through a tea strainer. If necessary, add cooled boiled water to replace the evaporated water up to original quantity.

5. Practical Advice for Six to Nine Months

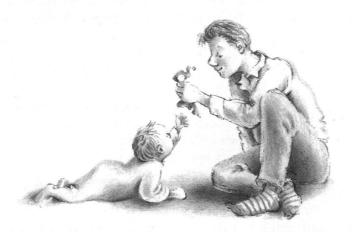

Psychomotor development

Now that the baby has gained control of his head, arms and trunk to some extent, he has a degree of freedom of movement. First, he discovers his feet as enjoyable toys. The child can experience his whole body from head to feet, though still with a rather dreamy consciousness. The child starts to move about, first by rolling over, and later on, at approximately nine months, by crawling.

During this stage, many children learn to raise themselves up into a stable sitting position. Some children move about on their front or shift themselves on their backsides, another method of exploring space.

The child's sounds can start to incorporate words such as gaga, dada or baba.

During this stage, the child learns to distinguish between familiar people — usually the mother and father, and others. It is typical of this stage for the baby to start to cling to a particular person, and seek security with those people to whom he is most attached.

Sleeping and waking

The pattern of sleeping and waking still largely follows the pattern of feeding. There are usually four meals in the day, at seven and eleven o'clock in the morning, and at three and seven o'clock in the afternoon and evening.

Most children still like to have a nap after the first and second feeds. The nap between three in the afternoon and seven o'clock gradually becomes shorter or disappears altogether. Many children like to be put in bed for a while, even if they do not sleep. For children who do not like this, the day is often just a little bit too long, which means they start to grizzle by teatime. In this case, try to give the seven o'clock feed slightly earlier. Most children will now sleep through the night.

Care

Washing and bathing

At this age it is not really necessary to bath the baby with soap every day. However, when a child starts to crawl on the floor, it is important to devote extra attention to hygiene.

Many children catch colds during the crawling stage because the floor is cold and there is often a draught close to the ground. Children cannot blow their noses at this age, so treat the face with an oily ointment such as calendula baby cream, so that the skin does not dry out too much.

The playpen

As the baby's freedom of movement and exploratory drive increases, it is quite an art to arrange the time spent in the playpen and outside to meet the child's needs. The playpen provides support for sitting and standing up, and gives the child an opportunity to examine and discover toys in a quiet place. Outside the playpen, the big world beckons, and the child is able to roll over and crawl about freely.

Do not put too many toys in the playpen, but make sure they are regularly changed. It is often useful to have a bag hanging from the wooden rungs to put the toys in. The baby should play with other toys outside the playpen, as this will increase the attraction of being put back in the playpen.

Toys and playing

When the child is in the playpen, he will not just look at and explore the toys, he will also use them. For example, he will hit a ball so that it rolls away, or grab hold of a rattle and hit it against the rungs of the playpen. The child can use any objects which are used for his daily care, such as a soap dish or flannel, or a spoon and beaker, provided they are safe.

Playing with adults, the child really enjoys games which involve moving, such as 'horsey games' or 'Round and round the garden.'

Once the child is crawling, the voyages of discovery really expand; it feels everything around it and often hits things with a flat hand. The child likes to hold something in his hand when crawling, and a wooden spoon or a lid of a jam jar can be used to make surprising sounds, for example, by hitting it on a wooden or tiled floor.

Every crumb, piece of fluff, bead or pin will be carefully picked up from the floor with the thumb and index finger and put into the mouth. Therefore it is important to pay attention to what is left on the floor, and remove anything that is dangerous.

Safety

The most common accidents during this period are caused by falls, knocks and bumps, burns, poisoning, drowning, strangulation and suffocation. Take the following precautions.

Falls

— From the dressing table, out of the high chair and the pram. Make sure that the chair or pram is stable and use a harness.
— From the stairs; install stair gates at the top and bottom of the stairs.

Knocks/bumps

— If necessary, place protective corners on sharp edges and points.

Burns/poisoning

— Keep hot drinks out of the child's way; use place mats rather that a tablecloth, so that baby cannot pull hot drinks and food over himself if he pulls on the tablecloth; make sure that electric cables are out of reach, for example; for a kettle.
— Make sure that toxic substances and plants, or any stray ashtray are kept out of the way.

Drowning

— **Never** leave the baby in the bath on his own, and place an anti-slip mat on the bottom of the bath.

Strangulation/suffocation

— Do not use a clamp to keep the blankets in place, or a harness in bed. However, many children no longer want to lie down in bed once they have learnt to stand up. This can lead to great drama at bedtime, and indicates that it is now time to lower the cot mattress. Use a baby's sleeping bag or make a warm overall, and make sure that the side of the bed is high enough so that the baby cannot fall out. If necessary, discuss this with the baby clinic.
— Once a baby reveals a tendency to stand up, remove everything from the playpen which could lead to strangulation or with which the child could hang himself; lines stretched across the playpen are also dangerous. Cords for Venetian blinds pose

a very real risk and should be tied up out of reach.

A number of the safety measures described here apply for children who can sit or stand up. Because of the safety aspect, these situations are discussed at this stage, although many babies do not sit or stand up until the next stage, between nine and twelve months.

Feeding

During this stage, the feeding pattern does not usually change very much. Usual feeding times are on waking, late morning, during the afternoon and early evening (see also Sleeping and waking, pp.69f).

However, there is a change in the actual diet. Often, breastfeeding comes to an end during this period, there is more variation in vegetables and fruit, and cereals and sour milk products such as live yoghurt can be introduced. A general diet could be as follows:

On waking
breastfeeding or bottle-feeding or porridge

Late morning
vegetables + cereals + pudding (breastfeeding, bottle or sour milk products)

Afternoon
fruit (+ cereal flakes) combined with breastfeeding, bottle-feeding or dairy products.

Early evening
breastfeeding or bottle-feeding or porridge

Breastfeeding

At the start of this stage, many babies are still breastfed four times a day. When the sucking reflex diminishes, two of the feeds can be dropped, that is, at 11am and 3pm. Gradually, the morning and evening feeds can be replaced with a bottle or with porridge.

When you want to stop feeding, you should gradually reduce the number of feeds. The pressure and the increased chance of mastitis often determine the rate at which you stop. It takes approximately five days to stop one feed. When you stop the last feed, it is not necessary to wait until the breasts are completely empty. When you no longer feel the milk coming in, you can stop feeding. Any milk that remains will be assimilated by the body.

Bottle-feeding

For bottle-feeding with bottles that you prepare yourself, you should now use the following ingredients:

Flour, milk, water, sweetener and cold-pressed sunflower or olive oil. At this age it is no longer necessary to add almond paste. The quantity can always be found on the packaging of the type of flour that was chosen. The milk is still diluted.

In our opinion, it is not necessary to give healthy children next stage milk rather than cow's milk (see also p.40).

Note: The instructions on some baby cereals state that the (diluted) milk should be cooked with the flour. It is better to boil the flour in enough water to produce a sort of paste, and then add the milk. Make sure that the baby gets 450 to 500 ml (½ quart) of milk products per day, if necessary, by adding some extra sour milk products (also see Weaning below).

Porridge

Porridge which is eaten with a spoon can be made with cereal flakes or flour.

The advantage of porridge made of cereal flakes is that you can vary these with different flakes and the child becomes used to a coarser type of porridge. Furthermore, cereal flakes are cheaper than flour. Buy the flakes in small quantities at a time so that they are always fresh.

Flakes which are suitable (in order from easily digestible flakes to slightly more difficult to digest flakes) include rice, buckwheat, millet, oat and barley flakes. Oat flakes have a laxative effect and sometimes give the baby a red bottom.

Porridge made with cereal flakes

1. Soak the flakes for thirty minutes (or longer) in a small but sufficient amount of water.
2. Bring the flakes in the water to the boil, stirring all the time with a wooden spoon.
3. Leave the flakes to soak for twenty or thirty minutes with the lid on

the pan on the hob or to warm in a pan of hot water (au bain marie). You can also leave the flakes to soak overnight in a preheated thermos flask (with a wide mouth).
4. Place the pan on a low heat and add milk at a temperature of approximately 60°C (140°F), stirring with a whisk. Leave the porridge to soak with the lid on the pan, off the heat for about fifteen minutes.
5. Liquidize the porridge if needed.
6. Sweeten the porridge with unrefined sugar, baby malt, rice or barley malt syrup or maple syrup, approximately one teaspoon per bowl.

No quantities are given for the preparation of the porridge made of cereal flakes. The total quantity per bowl is approximately 200 ml (7 fl oz). After a while, you will know exactly how much you need of all the different sorts of flakes to prepare porridge of the right consistency. Experience and a good quality pan also contribute greatly to the success of your porridge.

Weaning

Vegetables

The composition of the vegetables is two thirds cooked vegetables to one third cooked cereal flakes and one teaspoon of cold-pressed sunflower or olive oil. Altogether make 150 to 200 ml (5–7 fl oz) of puréed vegetables, or if they are soft and prepared with cereal flakes, they can be mashed. You can also add a teaspoon of almond paste to the vegetables to give it a richer mixture.

When the baby has got used to the vegetables mentioned for three to six months (see p.66), you can start to vary them with other vegetables. A summary of vegetables is included again on p.75 to show the possibilities.

The vegetables are shown in the order of the ease with which they can be digested, from those, which are easy to digest to those which are more difficult. The vegetables marked with an asterix (*) are rich in nitrates and should not be given more than twice a week. However, they do not have to be left out of the diet altogether as they make a healthy change from the other vegetables.

Flakes

The flakes which were mentioned above (p.73) for the porridge can also be added to the vegetables. To prepare them, follow the recipe for the porridge with cereal flakes up to step 4. If you like, you can also prepare the flakes for two days and keep them in the fridge.

Tip: If you have little time, you can also add instant cereals used for bottle-feeding to the green vegetables.

Dessert

If the baby is not breast or bottle fed after the vegetables, a dessert made of dairy products can complete the meal.

Types of dairy products

Give approximately 100 ml live yoghurt or approximately 40 ml of curds, diluted with water. It can be sweetened with concentrated apple or pear juice, maple syrup, or rice or barley malt syrup. Curds are diluted because they contain two to three times as many proteins as full-fat milk.

Fruit

The fruit consists of puréed fruit with cereal flakes, which may or may not be combined with some dairy products. Again the ratio is $^2/_3$ fruit to $^1/_3$ flakes (together 100–150 ml, 3–5 fl oz), supplemented to 150–200 ml (5–7 fl oz) with sour milk products.

Types of fruit

Apple, pear, tangerine, blueberry, raspberry, blackberry, peach, orange.

In moderation: strawberry, plum, and banana, as these might lead to a hypersensitive reaction or influence bowel movements.

Bread

Your child can start to eat bread from about eight months. To get used to it, give the baby a crust to munch and gnaw on, closely supervised. From nine months, when the child can sit on his own, he can also start to join you at the table to eat bread.

Root	Stem/leaves	Flower/fruit
carrot *beetroot Jerusalem artichoke parsnip	cauliflower *spinach *endive *lettuce *salad greens *leaf beet *fennel *kohlrabi *lamb's lettuce *pak choi	broccoli pumpkin courgette peas french beans runner beans mangetout fruit

All vegetables are cooked. Green vegetables can be added to the carrot, pumpkin etc. when it is nearly done, and cooked with it for a short while.

* Vegetables rich in nitrates; do not give more than twice a week.

6. Practical Advice for Nine to Twelve Months

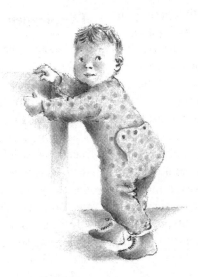

Psychomotor development

Once the child has learnt to crawl, the next stage is when she starts standing up. Often, a child of nine to ten months will start by standing on her knees, holding onto to the bars of the playpen. From ten or eleven months, she may be able to stand on her own feet, supported by the playpen or a chair. This is a great triumph! Statistically, the age of twelve months is characterized by the first independent steps. Often the child has already taken steps holding on to her parent's hand during the previous months. Therefore a one-year-old child has a (vague) awareness of her own body for the first time and is also able to start relating freely to space and gravity.

In fact, it is important to remember that the development described here in stages is based on averages. Virtually no child follows these statistics. Some children are faster, others slower. Sometimes a child will do something, which 'should' happen later, or will miss out a certain stage. This should not usually be a cause for concern. If you have any worries, discuss them at the baby clinic with the health visitor.

Apart from clinging to one person, the child may now also start to become frightened of separation. She will be aware of her mother moving away for a minute and will start to cry. At night, this can give rise to sleeping problems.

Sleeping and waking

At the beginning of this period, the rhythm of sleeping and waking is usually the same as for the previous period. By the end of the first year, many children are only taking one nap a day in the daytime.

This transition can be a difficult period, with a loss of the familiar pattern for both the child and parents. The child is too small for one nap and too big for two. It may be a month or more before a new pattern is established, both with regard to the nap, and with regard to feeding times.

Care

Brushing teeth

It is advisable to start brushing the child's teeth during this stage, once she has teeth, although you cannot expect too much of this at first. Choose a soft brush for your child and brush her teeth, or let her do this herself. If your child absolutely refuses to have her teeth brushed, this may be because of painful gums because teeth are still coming through.

Regularly brush your own teeth in the presence of your child and she will follow your good example. In our opinion, it is not necessary to use toothpaste at this stage. After brushing the teeth, give the child a sip of water, as this also cleans out the mouth.

The playpen

By about nine months, when the child is standing and crawling, the urge to explore the whole world is often so great that she will reject the playpen as a frustrating restriction. If you manage to persevere at that moment, you will benefit a great deal in the next few months. A safe place can then be guaranteed for at least one or two hours per day and that is a great advantage in a period when the child is sleeping less and is increasingly active, able to reach almost everything and throw things about.

When a child suddenly stops being a baby, the parents may find they have problems with upbringing that were inconceivable only a month before. Should I forbid this, should I punish my child if she touches the plants, or tears the covers off the books? The playpen imposes a clear boundary for the child and means that for while, you don't have to impose this boundary yourself.

In the playpen, the child learns to play with whatever is there at the time. This limitation means that it often plays in a more concentrated way than outside the playpen, where the range of interesting objects is so much larger.

Another advantage of the playpen is that other children in the family can play undisturbed for at least a few moments during the day, for example, without their wonderful tower of bricks being knocked over when it is only four bricks high.

It is obvious that outside the playpen the child also needs the space to learn to crawl and walk. Use the playpen at set times, for example, in the morning after breakfast, and in the afternoon while you are cooking dinner. Some children are satisfied in the playpen if their father or mother remains in sight. Other children will only play, after an initial protest, when there is no one in the room (though within hearing).

Sleeping problems

As indicated above, sleeping problems may arise during this stage. Children do not want to go to sleep at night or wake up crying several times during the night. The child must learn to feel confident that even if she cannot see her parents, they are still near by. They demand confirmation of this again and again. One thing which can give the child this confidence is a good bedtime routine, leaving the door slightly ajar with the light on in the corridor, with her own doll with a familiar odour, or sleeping with a brother or sister in the same room.

If there are problems with going to sleep, check whether the child is sleeping too much during the daytime or has been playing too many games before bedtime so that she is wide awake in the evening. Sometimes a bath can be helpful to calm the child down.

If a child cries at night, do not take her out of her own room, but try and calm her down by stroking her head or humming a lullaby.

Solving the sleeping problems by allowing the child to sleep in her parents' bed will probably lead to greater problems in the long run; that is, the child will only sleep there and will no longer sleep in her own bed.

Toys and playing

When the child can sit up on her own at the age of eight or nine months, she will be able to put things into a box or basket from this position. An old-fashioned toy box can be very useful for things to disappear into, such as bricks and cotton reels.

When the child starts to cling to certain people, this is the moment at which she first becomes aware that she is actually separate from the world. Playing 'Peekaboo' helps the child to realize unconsciously that you are there, even if she cannot see you. It gives a sense of confidence that there are always loving people around it.

Sitting in the high chair, the child will discover that when you drop something it suddenly goes a long way away or can no longer be seen. She also discovers that different objects make different sounds when they fall on the floor. This is such a fascinating experience, that the child cannot easily stop doing this by herself. At a certain point, you will have to indicate that enough is enough; for example, by no longer picking the object up.

Towards the end of the first year, we see that the child imitates everything that is happening around her: she likes to stir a spoon around a bowl when she sees father or mother doing this. Or she wants to eat by herself because older brothers or sisters do.

Safety

The most common accidents are the same as those described for six to nine months. However, during this stage, the child starts moving about more and can do much more, so that the risks increase. Impose clear boundaries with the use of stair gates, harnesses in the high chair, and the playpen. Make sure you have an age-appropriate car seat, or if you cycle, a safe bicycle seat and cycle helmet. Adapt the situation in the house to this age by placing dangerous or vulnerable objects out of reach or putting them away. Give the child her own shelf or cupboard where she can do her own thing. Always remove the child from places where she can be 'naughty.' Forbidding anything at this age is pointless. Make sure that there are no loose objects around the child, that she could choke on; marbles, beads and nuts are a common source of danger.

Feeding

During this stage a child often clearly indicates that she wants to join in. At this age, this means that she wants to enjoy the domestic togetherness at the table even though she does not have to eat the same food as the others yet.

Therefore, times have been left out in the summary of meals given below and the meals are indicated as breakfast, dinner, etc. However, lunch is usually much earlier than the time lunch is normally eaten because this is more suitable for the sleeping pattern.

Breakfast: a bowl of porridge and some bread and drinking from a beaker if necessary.
Possibly a snack in between meals with a drink.
Lunch: vegetables and dairy pudding
Teatime: fruit and possibly a drink
Dinner: porridge and some bread and a drink if necessary.

During this period, the bottle usually gradually disappears from the scene. Porridge is eaten from a bowl and the baby can often manage to drink from a beaker quite successfully.

Porridge

You can give the porridge or cereal flakes, described for six to nine months (see p.73) or prepare porridge with flour.

Bread

This is the age at which a child often starts to chew. If she has few or no teeth, she will do so with her gums. Therefore, the child can start to chew its bread, rather than merely sucking on it as in the previous stage. To eat a real sandwich, it is important for a child to sit up so that she does not choke so easily. The bread will gradually replace the porridge, though usually not before the first year. At first, bread is a good way to introduce food which can be chewed. Start with light brown bread and go on to wholemeal bread at about one year.

Spreads

Unsalted butter, nut paste (if no parents with a nut allergy), cream cheese and fruit compote.

Peanuts are not nuts, but pulses. Therefore it is best to not give peanut butter. It is heavier to digest and leads more often to allergies than nuts do (see Pulses, pp.43f).

Drinking

As the food becomes more solid the child needs extra drinks, particularly when the weather is hot. However, the total amount of moisture per day should not be more than one litre / quart.

Herbal tea, fruit juice or apple juice are suitable drinks. However, try to prevent a one-sided pattern from developing, for example, only giving apple juice. Large amounts of juice should be avoided because of the sugar content. Milk does not quench thirst, but is a form of food. Whether you give milk with a meal depends on the rest of the eating pattern; a child needs about 450 to 500 ml (about half a quart) of dairy products per day.

Bottles

Some children will not be parted from their bottle. They would like to drink all day if possible. We advise that you do not give into this because drinking too much diminishes the appetite. This applies particularly if you give squash or another such drink.

Drinking sweet juice from a bottle can also lead to problems if the child develops a sweet tooth, and can lead to dental decay in the front teeth. In our view, using a beaker with a spout as a transition from the bottle to the beaker is not desirable, because the child may want to suck on this all day. It is best is to go from a bottle directly to a normal cup, because this is best for the mouth muscles in relation to speech development.

Snacks

Suitable snacks are toast or crisp-baked biscuits, a crust of bread,

Ryvita, rice cakes, bread sticks. Never give the child these snacks without supervision because of the danger of choking.

Vegetables

The vegetables can be mashed or cut up more coarsely. Instead of adding oil you can also add some butter or cream to the vegetables. The flakes can be alternated with wholemeal macaroni or spaghetti.

It is still too early for whole grain rice, barley etc.

Fruit

The fruit should be sufficiently nutritious to help the child get through the afternoon. On the other hand, it should not be so filling that it takes away the child's appetite for dinner. Therefore, depending on the child, it could consist of puréed fruit with or without flakes and/or dairy products.

7. Aspects of Care for the Small Child

Tests, vitamins and development

The PKU and CHT test

Depending on where you live, the midwife, health visitor, obstetrician or sometimes your doctor will visit between the fifth and the seventh day after the birth to give the child a 'heel test.'

A few drops of blood are collected from a small prick in the heel. This blood is examined for PKU (*phenylketonuria,* a metabolic disorder) and CHT (an adrenal hormone, of which there may be a deficiency). Both these rare diseases can cause brain damage, but can be treated at an early stage through diet and medicines respectively.

Make sure that the baby's feet are warm for the prick in the heel. This makes it easier to take blood.

Vitamin K

In recent years, parents have been advised to give babies extra vitamin K. The advice applies to the period that the body does not produce suffi-cient vitamin K itself, that is, during the first three months. The aim is to prevent some babies from developing serious — and in some cases fatal — bleeding (for example, in the brain). These cases are extremely rare and are attributed to slow coagulation of the blood, a complicated system with many different 'coagulation factors.' By giving vitamin K, the aim is to accelerate the development of the coagulating mechanism and thus reduce the chance of bleeding.

In a number of countries, including the UK, a vitamin K injection is usually administered to newborn babies immediately after birth. An alternative option, is to give vitamin K orally at birth, followed by further doses on days 4 to 7, and a third dose at one month.

In our opinion, there is a great deal to be said for giving a breast-fed child extra vitamin K for the first three months, in view of the seriousness of the complications concerned, the small amounts of the vitamin given for an extremely short period, and the absence of side effects.

Vitamin D and rickets

Nowadays, rickets is mostly a serious problem among immigrant populations. Rickets can be seen as a disease in which the body is not sufficiently connected with the earth. This is expressed in a developmental disorder and problems with calcium, particularly in the skeletal structure. The 'earthly' character of the body is related to the development of bones and calcifying processes. These processes give the body a more solid character and also help it to develop. For example, the late appearance or non-appearance of teeth or a slow motor development in the case of rickets can be 'made up' at an accelerated rate with the help of vitamin D.

However, in children who would not get rickets, the vitamin D stimulates accelerated development under normal circumstances. These children mature earlier and are therefore also intellectually stimulated. You must make a conscious choice whether you want this or not, because accelerated development is not always harmless. It can take vital forces from the body, which are really needed for the body to develop over a longer period. Therefore giving vitamin D as a matter of course does not seem desirable.

However, devoting attention to preventing rickets is important for all children. How rickets can be prevented must be determined by the doctor at the baby clinic for each child individually.

Rickets can be prevented by ensuring there is enough contact with sunlight and outside air or by giving vitamin D.

Therefore it is a good idea for the child to spend at least an hour and half per day in direct contact with the outside air or with daylight. This is even possible in autumn, winter and spring, whatever the weather, in a pram that has been heated with hot water bottles and removed before the child is placed inside.

Children with dark skin are at greater risk, and the doctor at the health centre should keep an eye on them.

Vitamin D is added to formula milk as a standard supplement; therefore, this will have to be taking into account when you are making a choice.

In some countries all children are checked for symptoms of rickets at the baby clinic, or at least, an attempt is made to do so. It is advisable to be aware of the vitamin D policy and to discuss it with a doctor at the baby clinic. Although it is a rare disease, rickets can have a number of unpleasant symptoms, which are not always predictable. It is also difficult to predict who is and who is not susceptible to rickets.

This makes it more difficult to adopt an individual policy. Nevertheless it is worth trying to do so.

Development of the teeth — fluoride

It looks so ordinary, but is actually quite extraordinary. We are born without visible teeth. During the course of the first three years, the milk teeth appear, and at the age of about six, the teeth simply fall out to be replaced with the permanent teeth. These permanent teeth and molars are only formed after birth.

It is quite remarkable that this development can indicate the actual state of the development of the organism as a whole. At birth, the 'milk organism' is still unfinished to a great extent; it needs time to develop. In addition, the whole organism must be transformed in the first seven years to produce a permanent organism.

Because of their enamel, teeth are the hardest organs we possess, and are harder than bone. When the milk teeth appear — a process that takes place on average between the ages of six months and two and a half years — it marks the development of a weak, not very robust baby into a toddler with an independent relationship to space, and his first independent thought processes.

We have already seen that the sense of self and starting to use the word 'I,' only appear when the child has learnt to walk, talk and think (p.20); it is fascinating to see that the development of the teeth takes place in parallel with this. Perhaps it is understandable: the hard crystalline elements that form the teeth are formed under the influence of very specific forces, and these forces are released when they have completed their task.

In the anthroposophical view of the human being there is a connection between the forces which are released to form the teeth and 'earthly' thought processes. Earthly thinking refers to the clear 'solid' thought processes, which are more or less strongly developed in adults, but are completely absent in a newborn child. A child can only develop this way of thinking when the body, and in particular the milk teeth, have developed to some extent.

One problem which affects virtually everyone nowadays is *caries;* that is, holes in the teeth. The hard enamel dissolves because bacteria in the plaque on the teeth produce acid. Scientists have discovered that giving fluoride in the form of tablets, toothpaste or as a coating, can harden the enamel and therefore help to prevent caries.

Fluoride is found naturally in the teeth enamel, and in the bones. It has a binding, formative effect, inhibiting life forces and hardening the tissues.

Dentine, the tissue under the enamel is a very different substance. Its main element is magnesium, which has the effect of stimulating life, and is also found in the green leaves of plants.

In the development of the teeth, the relationship between magnesium and fluoride plays an important role. Naturally, the proportion of magnesium is 32 times greater than fluoride in the teeth, which indicates how unbelievably powerful the effect of fluoride is, and explains why too much fluoride is unnatural and therefore not required.

These days, attention is paid above all to the hardening substance which inhibits life, fluoride. Because of concern regarding caries, it is understandable that all children are advised to have fluoride. Fluoride certainly does prevent the appearance of caries, but what else does it do?

On the basis of the *relationship* described above between enamel (fluoride) and dentine (magnesium), it is understandable that too much flouride in the dentine can actually have a harmful effect because the magnesium should predominate. In fact, one of the side-effects of taking fluoride for years can be damage to the dentine.

However, fluoride also has an effect on the subtle link between the forces which form and harden the teeth and the development of the thought processes. By giving fluoride to young children the hardening processes are strengthened and accelerated throughout the whole body. This reinforcement of physical hardening also leads to an acceleration in the psychological development of the child; it encourages a premature development in the thoughts and feelings. One of the consequences of this is that the child is 'awake' to the world at an earlier age.

With a good diet, fluoride supplementation is unneccessary. Moreover, fluoride influences the movements of the gut in a negative way. So we do not recommend supplementing fluoride in toothpaste or otherwise.

What can you do to prevent caries if you do not want to give fluoride?

Obviously diet (wholemeal products and small quantities of sweet products), learning to chew well, and oral hygiene all play a role. When the first teeth appear, it is a good idea to brush them with a soft toothbrush. Shortly after drinking fruit juice you should not brush your teeth, but clean them with a sip of water. In our view, toothpaste is not really necessary (see also p.78). From the age of two and a half it is advisable to go to the dentist regularly.

It is important to be aware of the relationship between magnesium and fluoride processes. For example, who are generally wide awake and alert, have their small teeth sooner under the influence of fluoride, while children who are rather dreamy often have large teeth as a result of the effect of the magnesium. In fact, both types of children can develop caries. It may be useful to support the development of the teeth with the help of anthroposophical medication on the advice of an anthroposophical doctor or dentist. The magnesium processes can be reinforced in the diet by giving green vegetables no more than twice a week (because of the nitrate content, see pp.74f).

In summary, it can be said that the development of the teeth is an expression of the whole of the child's development, and that fluoride plays a role in this, though not the *only* role. Brushing with fluoride toothpaste accelerates the hardening processes.

Vaccinations

As the parent of a newborn child, you will inevitably be confronted with the issue of vaccinations. It is possible to vaccinate against a whole range of contagious or infectious diseases. Some of these infectious diseases are also known as the traditional childhood diseases. Every parent has a free choice with regard to vaccination.

The infectious diseases for which there are vaccinations are listed below with a description of the advantages and disadvantages of vaccinating, and what the possible alternatives might be. Because of a lack of space, the information provided here cannot be complete. However, we hope that a considered choice can be made in consultation

with the doctor with regard to vaccinations, on the basis of the information and the vision given here, and with the recommended additional information. If your child should catch an infectious disease, always contact your doctor. Supportive treatment for different infectious diseases exists in anthroposophical medicine.

Infectious diseases

In most countries, the immunization programme is comprised of vaccines against the following diseases: diptheria, tetanus, whooping cough (pertussis), polio, haemophilus influenza type B (Hib), as well as maningitis and later measles, mumps and German measles (rubella). The programme varies in different countries and is regularly revised. There is an overview on p.90.

Whooping cough, mumps, measles and German measles are known as the traditional childhood diseases. We will briefly mention the cause of the disease, the symptoms, the possible complications (which may appear but do not appear in all cases), the possible treatments and the protection provided by the vaccine.

Diphtheria

Diphtheria is a bacterial infection transmitted by coughing. The disease mainly affects the area around the nose, throat and larynx, and can result in loss of breath and even suffocation. The disease can cause permanent damage to the heart, kidneys and nervous system, and the death rate is very high. The diphtheria vaccine provides total protection against this disease. The vaccination is usually given at 8, 12 and 16 weeks of age as part of a combined DTP or 5-in-1 inoculation.

Whooping cough (pertussis)

Whooping cough is an extremely contagious, bacterial, infectious disease, which is transmitted by coughing. The coughing fits usually occur at night and continue for about six weeks. After a coughing fit, the child usually goes back to sleep straightaway, and may be lively and cheerful during the daytime. However, it can be a very tiring period, particularly for parents.

In children under the age of one, there may be complications with periods when the child stops breathing, resulting in brain damage. The long and forceful coughing can also damage the lungs, and lead to middle ear infections. Complications rarely occur in children over the age of one. At an early stage, whooping cough can be treated with antibiotics. However, at that stage, it is not easy to tell whether the illness is a case of whooping cough or simply a bad cold.

The vaccination is usually given at 8, 12 and 16 weeks of age as part of a combined DTP or 5-in-1 inoculation. After being vaccinated, some children still get whooping cough, though usually in a milder form.

Tetanus (lockjaw)

It is possible to be infected with tetanus as a result of all sorts of injuries, as the tetanus bacteria are found in many places, indoors and outdoors. This disease is characterized by vehement muscular cramps including cramp in the respiratory muscles. The disease is difficult to treat and the death rate is very high.

The tetanus vaccine provides complete protection against the disease. The vaccination is usually given at 8, 12 and 16 weeks of age as part of a combined DTP or 5-in-1 inoculation.

Polio (infantile paralysis)

Polio is caused by a virus, and is passed on through the faeces of an infected person. In general, the disease is fairly harmless, accompanied only by diarrhea, but in a small percentage of people it causes permanent damage to the nervous and motor systems. As in the case of other viral infections, there is no regular medication, such as an antibiotic, for polio. The vaccination is usually given at 8, 12 and 16 weeks of age, sometimes as part of a combined 5-in-1 inoculation.

Hib diseases

These concern serious, fairly common, bacterial infectious diseases, which are particularly prevalent amongst young children. The Hib bacteria are transmitted by coughing and sneezing and can result in a type of meningitis, swelling of the epiglottis and inflammation of the joints. The disease has acute symptoms and sometimes results in permanent damage, such as deafness, epilepsy and brain damage, though rarely resulting in death. The disease can be treated with antibiotics, but as it usually develops very rapidly it is not always possible to treat it adequately.

The vaccine protects the child against all Hib diseases, but not against other forms of meningitis such as meningitis C (see below). The vaccination is usually given at 8, 12 and 16 weeks of age, sometimes as part of a combined 5-in-1 inoculation.

Pneumococci

As with Hib, this type of meningitis apperars most frequently in the first few months of life. As well as meningitis, pneumococci can also cause middle ear infections and pneumonia. The strain of pneumoccocus often varies from country to country and so vaccines tend to be country-specific. The vaccination is usually given at 8, 12 and 16 weeks of age.

Meningitis C

Many people carry this bacteria without any ill effects. In rare cases it may lead to meningitis and septicaemia. First indications are similar to symptoms of flu but it quickly develops into a serious illness with high fever, and can lead to disorientation and lethargy. Other symptoms include headaches, stiffness of the neck, severe headache at the front of the head and possibly a small, pimply rash. If symptoms appear, seek immediate medical advice.

The vaccination is usually given at 12 and 16 weeks of age.

Mumps

Mumps is a viral disease and is transmitted by coughing. Mumps is accompanied by an inflammation of the salivary gland, located below each ear. Some rare and, in general, harmless complications include meningitis and inflammation of the pancreas. If this disease occurs after puberty, this occasionally has an effect on the testicles in boys, and the ovaries in girls, leading to problems with fertility in very rare cases. Deafness is another fairly rare complication.

The mumps vaccine provides almost complete protection against the mumps, and is often given from the age of 12 months onwards as part of the 3-in-1 MMR vaccine.

Measles

Measles is a viral disease and is transmitted by coughing and sneezing. In the initial stages, the disease is like a sort of flu with coughing and the symptoms of a cold. After that the measles really take hold and the child will feel very ill. Some of the complications that can be treated include middle ear infection and pneumonia. A low level of resistance, and giving fever suppressants,

Gov't recommended immunization	UK	Ireland	USA	Can	Aus	NZ	SAfrica
Birth							
BCG tuberculosis		x					x
hepatitis B			x		x		
polio							x
6–8 weeks							
diphtheria, tetanus, pertussis*	5in1	5in1	DTP	DTP	DTP	DTP	DTP
polio	5in1	5in1	IPV	IPV	IPV	IPV	x
Hib	5in1	5in1	x	x	x	x	x
hepatitis B			x		x	x	x
meningitis C		x		x			
pneumococci	x		x	x	x		
3–4 months							
diphtheria, tetanus, pertussis*	5in1	5in1	DTP	DTP	DTP	DTP	DTP
polio	5in1	5in1	IPV	IPV	IPV	IPV	x
Hib	5in1	5in1	x	x	x	x	x
hepatitis B			x		x	x	x
meningitis C	x	x					
pneumococci			x	x	x		
4–6 months							
diphtheria, tetanus, pertussis*	5in1	5in1	DTP	DTP	DTP	DTP	DTP
polio	5in1	5in1		IPV	IPV	IPV	x
Hib	5in1	5in1		x	x		x
hepatitis B					x	x	x
meningitis C	x	x		x			
pneumococci	x		x	x	x		
9 months							
measles							measles
12–18 months							
diphtheria, tetanus, pertussis*			DTP	DTP			DTP
polio			IPV	IPV			x
Hib	x	x	x	x	x	x	
hepatitis B			x				
measles, mumps, rubella	MMR	MMR	MMR	MMR	MMR	MMR	measles
meningitis C	x				x		
pneumococci	x		x	x			
varicella			x	x			
chickenpox					x		

pertussis = whooping cough

See page 119 for websites of government recommendations

can increase the chance of these complications. The complication of encephalitis can cause serious permanent damage or even be fatal, although this is extremely rare. The vaccine provides complete protection against the disease, and is often given from the age of 12 months onwards as part of the 3-in-1 MMR vaccine.

German measles (rubella)

German measles is a viral disease, which is fairly harmless in children. The symptoms include a red rash, swollen glands in the neck and a raised temperature. German measles can cause defects in an unborn child, especially during the first few months of pregnancy.

The vaccine provides virtually complete protection against the disease, and is often given from the age of 12 months onwards as part of the 3-in-1 MMR vaccine.

Other vaccinations

There are also a number of vaccinations which are only given in special cases; for example, to specific at-risk groups owing to family history, country of origin or in instances of chronic disease. These include vaccinations against tuberculosis and flu.

In time, the general range of vaccinations will probably be extended even further. At the moment, research is being carried out into the possibilities of vaccinating against certain types of meningitis (other than those caused by the Hib bacteria).

Most countries do not vaccinate against illnesses such as chicken pox (apart from the USA and Canada), because they are very mild and there are few complications.

Most vaccination programmes include vaccines against diseases which hardy occur anymore in the developed world. The reason for keeping these vaccines in use is the belief that they will certainly return if no vaccinations are given against these diseases.

The principle of inoculation

The vaccines used to inoculate children contain traces of the disease concerned. However, these traces have been altered in a laboratory, and have either been killed or weakened so that they can no longer give rise to all the symptoms of the disease. Therefore, the inoculated child receives the disease in a very weak, almost unnoticed form. This encourages the immune system to create antibodies against the disease for which the child was inoculated.

If the child then comes into contact with the disease at a later date, the immune system can deal with the infection straightaway so that the child will not catch the natural form of the disease.

Are the vaccinations compulsory?

Although many people think vaccinations are compulsory for children, this is not the case. However, some childcare centres for children require vaccinations as a condition for enrolment. It is advisable to ask for information about this in good time.

Side effects of vaccination

Just as there are complications with the infectious diseases described here, there can also be side effects resulting from the different vaccines. In the first place, there are harmless side effects, such as a slightly raised temperature, feeling unwell and redness in the place where the child was inoculated. In addition, some vaccines can lead to more violent reactions. There may be a high temperature, vomiting, long periods of crying, listlessness, irritability, fainting and convulsions. However, these symptoms are not considered to be a reason not to vaccinate the child concerned again, since the damage is not permanent.

However, some parents have also told stories about children who were never ill until they were vaccinated, and who then struggled with constant fevers and colds. An association which has carried out some critical research into vaccinations, particularly the side effects, has come to some different conclusions than the officials do, but is difficult

to prove scientifically. Ultimately, it is about parental choice.

If you want to make a considered choice with regard to vaccinations, we advise parents to read the vaccination booklets which are available from any health centre, as well as reading as widely as possible. The book, *Vaccination: A Guide for Making Personal Choices,* by Studer and Douch contains further information on this subject. *A Guide to Child Health* by Glöckler and Goebel has a thorough discussion on the pros and cons of each vaccine (see bibliography on p.117).

Practical tips

You should not let your child be inoculated if he has a fever or if you suspect that he is sickening for something. In principle, the common cold is not a reason not to have an inoculation.

From the day of the inoculation, and for a few days afterwards, the child may cry a lot, be unwell or ill and have a fever up to 40°C (104°F). The body has to assimilate the inoculation. Any extra rushing about, excitement, watching TV, going on a visit or on a trip etc, is not advisable during the days after a vaccination, nor is playing in bright sunlight. All this can be too much for the child.

If the place around the inoculation is red and painful, a piece of cloth soaked in cold water or with some curds can provide some relief. It is also possible to put some arnica 20% (Weleda) in the water to reduce swelling.

Immunity

When a child suffers from a number of the diseases described here he usually builds up a lifelong immunity. This applies particularly for the traditional childhood diseases, such as whooping cough, mumps, measles and German measles.

As a result of a vaccination, the child is given immunity against the disease for which he was inoculated. The question is whether there is a significant difference between the immunity acquired as a result of having the disease, and the immunity acquired as result of a vaccination. In our opinion, this question deserves attention and further research.

The question of the effects which inoculations have on the child's health in the longer term, is also raised increasingly frequently. There are indications that inoculating weakens, rather than strengthens, natural immunity, and it is not inconceivable that nature will create new manifestations of the disease if childhood diseases are otherwise eradicated. The many unidentified rashes and allergies which a large number of children suffer from nowadays point in this direction. The new variations may be worse than the original illness. It is possible to see the emergence of the many new allergic diseases in this light and possibly also the auto-immune diseases in which the body forms antibodies against parts of its own body.

The consequences of not vaccinating

When they progress normally, the diseases mentioned here are acute infectious diseases with a beginning, a peak and an end, which usually leave the child with lifelong immunity. With all childhood diseases, some children will be very ill, while others are hardly ill at all. It is also possible to acquire immunity without appearing to have the illness. It can happen that all the children in the family get a particular childhood disease, except for one child who does not catch it.

With all the diseases mentioned here, there can be complications, which mean that they do not progress in the normal way. The chances of this vary a great deal between the various childhood diseases. It is not possible to predict which child will suffer these abnormalities. This is what makes the decision about vaccinating so difficult.

Children who are not vaccinated still have a fairly high chance of catching certain childhood diseases. It is only when the child has caught one of these diseases that the consequences of not vaccinating become apparent. This brings a confrontation between feelings of guilt and the remarks and prejudices of other people. The consequences can be far-reaching; for example, the child can infect an adult, whose vaccination is no longer effective. It is impossible to anticipate all the consequences in advance. Is this then a reason to vaccinate? Or is it a reason *not* to vaccinate? There are not many situations in which you take decisions without being able to oversee all the consequences. On the basis of the information available at the moment, the examples you have seen around you, the practical considerations or the fear which you feel, you will make a decision and you cannot know how this will feel a month or a year later.

Perhaps it helps to know that a decision which has been taken with a great deal of thought gives support and confidence, and contributes to the future of the child in a positive way. And a decision taken consciously makes it more possible to deal with any disappointments resulting from that decision.

Alternative vaccination schedules

If you wish to change the time/age at which your child is vaccinated, there are other possibilities.

The chance of complications with whooping cough are greatest in the first year, and very slight afterwards. If you wish to vaccinate against whooping cough, it is thus advisable to do so in accordance with the usual schedule. The same applies for the Hib vaccination, as this relatively rare disease is most common during the first year.

If you choose not to vaccinate against whooping cough, it may be possible to start with individual vaccinations against diptheria, tetanus and polio later. In this case, the fist vaccinations would be given at 12 months, the second 4–6 weeks later, and a third one six months after that, at around 19 to 20 months. Altogether there would be one less booster because the immune system has developed much further.

It is also quite possible *not* to vaccinate against certain illnesses until after the childhood diseases, that is, between the ages of 12 and 14 for measles, mumps and German measles. This is because the possible complications of measles are more serious after the age of ten years.

Whatever you decide, it is important to discuss it thoroughly with your doctor. He or she will have to monitor your child when he is ill.

The purpose of illness and fever

The childhood diseases mentioned here are all accompanied by fever. A fever is the natural weapon of the organism to fight against germs. It is well known that viruses and bacteria cannot multiply very easily at temperatures over 39°C (102°F). A fever activates the immune system so that it will also be able to respond to germs appropriately in the future. In this sense, a fever helps the organism to develop a good immune system.

People are afraid of fever and often try to find ways to bring the fever down as quickly as possible. In our view, this fear of fever is unjustified, and by suppressing the fever, you prevent the organism from having a chance to build up a healthy resistance. Thus we see fever as a friend, rather than as a foe. On p.97, we look at practical ways of dealing with fever.

In general, it may be said that there are two sides to being ill. On the one hand, illness is a disturbing factor; it interrupts the normal course of events in life, causes pain, discomfort, sorrow, suffering, pressure on others, absenteeism and incurs costs.

On the other hand, you can also say that illness leads somewhere. Looking back at an illness, you often see that it did not appear out of nowhere, but that this was a decisive moment in life. In small ways, this can occur when you are exhausted, or in bigger ways, for example, when you have to make an important decision about your life. Sometimes, the actual illness can help to reveal a new path.

Does this also apply to the infectious diseases in childhood? From an anthroposophical point of view,

these diseases are essential helpers in the development of the child. How can this be explained?

Every child inherits certain physical characteristics from his parents. This is like a sort of home in which he will live throughout his life. During the first years of childhood, it is important to move into this 'home' fully, and make it his own, as it were.

Sometimes, certain aspects of this physicality do not appear to fit very well. The child can make use of the infectious diseases to transform or rebuild these aspects. They help him to transform his physicality in such a way that he 'fits' better. Obviously, this is a better starting position for exploring the world from one's own 'house' later on. In this way every infectious disease during childhood makes it possible to carry out a particular aspect of the 'conversion.' Parents often observe that after having had one of the childhood diseases, their children really have become 'better' and have not really returned to their old selves.

Therefore, an infectious disease gives a child the opportunity of conquering a particular developmental barrier at the physical level. Barriers which are not conquered have to be crossed in a different way after childhood, for example, through a process of self-education, and that is by no means always easy.

Common health problems

When should I consult a doctor?

No parent can avoid the difficult or anxious questions about their child's health, particularly when it is a first child. As adults, we are usually able to assess our own situation but how can you know about the sickness or health of a baby who doesn't say or indicate anything?

The guidelines given below can serve as an aid to finding your way around this 'unknown territory.' It should be remembered that these are general guidelines which do not always apply to a unique and specific situation.

Fever

When the body temperature is over 38°C (100.4°F) this constitutes a fever.

How high can the temperature be allowed to go? How long may the fever last? When can a fever be harmful?

These are common questions which indicate that fever is a source of anxiety, and which also reveal that fever is seen as an enemy. It may be surprising to hear that the doctor will not only be interested in exactly what the child's temperature is, but also in its general state; for example, a child with an appendicitis and a temperature of 38.5°C (101.3°F) is much more seriously ill than a child with a cold and a temperature of 40.4°C (104.7°F). Meningitis is not necessarily accompanied by a high temperature either, and yet it is a very serious disease. In fact, a fever is the way in which the organism combats the bacteria or virus; they are conquered by the heat.

Seen in this light, fever is more of a friend than a foe, and inhibiting the fever is not very sensible. The most important question when a child has a fever is whether it seems unwell. Is the child actually ill or actually quite well, but with a fever? It is certainly not easy to describe what is meant by 'really ill.'

For a child under one, the *level of consciousness* is very important; a child with fever may be sleepy, but it must be able to wake up. If a child is dozy and cannot really wake up, this is a bad sign.

Taking *liquids* is also very important. The smaller the child and the higher the fever, the more vulnerable the system is to dehydration. On the other hand, dehydration occurs virtually only with gastroenteritis (diarrhea and vomiting) with a fever. If there is no diarrhea, you can tell from the wet nappies how often the child is urinating; twice in 24 hours is an absolute minimum. If a child urinates more often, there is generally no question of dehydration. If you use disposable nappies, it is sometimes difficult to ascertain how much a child has urinated.

For the respiratory system, *coughing* and *breathlessness* are important symptoms. A small child who cannot breathe easily (except if it has a blocked nose) is obviously sick; coughing can originate in the lungs or in the mucus membranes of the nose. If a cough is a nuisance, leads to breathlessness or is persistent, it is necessary to consult a doctor.

Crying vehemently or for long periods can be a sign of pain. If a child with a cold and a fever cries particularly when it is put down, or suddenly and repeatedly wakes up crying, this is a probable sign of a middle ear infection. A middle ear infection is very painful, and it is good to use medicines for this in consultation with the doctor (see also earache, p.101).

Fevers are also common in the case of *gastroenteritis*, as indicated above If the baby only has diarrhea, it is good to give her extra liquids in addition to the adapted feeds. When a child throws everything up, it is pointless to give feeds or liquids; in this case, it is certainly a good idea to consult the doctor.

The most common situations in which a child has fever have been described above We have tried to explain that the accompanying symptoms are more important than the actual temperature. A fever in itself is never harmful, even if it is as high as 41.7°C (107°F), which seems to be about the highest possible fever. It is not possible to give a general rule about how long a fever might last. In a small child, it certainly seems sensible to consult a doctor if she has had a fever for three days, because of her vulnerability. If you are anxious, you can obviously consult the doctor earlier.

Many parents are afraid of *febrile convulsions*. Parents whose child has had such a convulsion once are particularly anxious because they are so frightening. A convulsion lasts a short while (maximum five minutes) and is an attack in which the child convulses and wholly, or partly, loses consciousness. The convulsion almost always occurs during a period when the fever is rising, as it is going up very quickly. Once the fever is at a high level, there is very little chance of a convulsion. A convulsion does not do any damage, and is not a sign of epilepsy. If the attack lasts longer than five minutes it may be necessary to consider epilepsy, and the child should be examined more thoroughly.

Convulsions occur up to the age of four years. Once a child has had a convulsion, she may have another convulsion the next time she has a fever, though this does not necessarily happen.

It is not a good idea to suppress the fever with fever suppressants. In fact, the chances are that the fever will actually go up again when the suppressant ceases to have an effect, and that this might lead to a convulsion.

One of the treacherous things is that during the first weeks after birth the child can actually respond to an infection with a very low temperature, instead of with a fever. This also reveals that it is not the temperature that is the important thing, but actually the child's condition.

When the child's condition requires this, for example, if she is delirious, it is a good idea to give her a lemon wrap (see procedure and illustration on p.111). The baby's trunk, and particularly the feet must be warm, also after the wrap. The fever will usually drop by half a degree as a result of the wrap. which can be removed after half an hour.

If there is no change in the baby's condition and her feet are still warm, you can prepare a new wrap. When the child is asleep, the wrap can simply be left in place.

Treating health problems in the first year

In general, it may be said that a sick child needs extra care, and that resting (in bed) is very important. If the carer feels confident about the way things are, and is not afraid of the situation, this will give the child a sense of security which will help her to get over the illness. It is not a good idea to bathe a child while she is ill, as the loss of temperature which results from this requires too much strength.

Immediately after birth, small problems may arise which can usually be treated with simple reme-

dies. If you do not trust the situation or do not know what to do, contact the nurse and/or doctor.

Stomach cramps (colic)

Between the ages of six weeks and three months, many children (one in six) suffer from stomach cramps (colic). The child cries loudly, bangs her head back and pulls up her legs. She likes to be held upright and carried around. Holding the baby firmly and wrapping her up warm in a blanket often helps her to relax. If this is not sufficient, swaddling is a tried and tested remedy (see p.29 and 108). Also keep a eye on your own stress level!

— A warm cloth with camomile oil (see p.111), some sieved camomile tea, or Weleda Baby and Child Bath in the bathwater can also have a relaxing effect.

— Some copper ointment on the stomach can help to treat the cramps. Apply the ointment with a warm hand, in rotating movements around the navel, in a clockwise direction.

— Fennel tea (see p.110) can help if you hear gurgling noises in the stomach and the child has a lot of wind.

If the child needs complete relaxation, a bath with camomile tea can be very restful. This bath should only be given if the child is not ill in any other way. It may be necessary to adapt the mother's diet in consultation with the nurse or baby clinic.

Blocked nose

Many newborn babies have a blocked nose. You can hear this because the baby makes a sort of grunting noise; drinking is more difficult because the baby has to take in air all the time and she keeps letting go of the breast or bottle.

You can give her some physiological saline drops. These are sold at the chemist, and if necessary, you can make them yourself by dissolving one teaspoon of salt in a glass of tepid water; place one drop in each nostril with a dropper before giving the feed. Never use cold water, as this is an unpleasant feeling for the child, and do not give any more because this will lead to too much salt in the stomach. Using mild nose balm (Wala), on and around the nose can also be helpful.

Sticky eyes

In the beginning, the eyes may become inflamed now and again with yellow crusts. Often the eyes are completely gummed up. This may be because the tear ducts are not yet open, and you cannot really do anything about this in the first year.

What you must do is to clean the eyes as soon as the child wakes up. This can be done by carefully rubbing the eye clean with a piece of cotton wool soaked in tepid camomile tea or cooled boiled water (camomile has disinfectant properties), and rubbing it from the outside in, towards the tearduct. Take a new piece of cotton wool every time you pass it across the eye.

White spots in the mouth

If there are white spots on the inside of the mouth which do not disappear, this is probably a case of thrush. It is advisable to clean the mouth after every feed with a cloth and some fungal inhibiting remedy. We mention a number of household remedies here. Depending on the seriousness of the complaint, it is possible to see whether the baby responds well to one or more of the following remedies:

— Molkosan (Vogel) diluted in a ratio of 1 to 4
— blueberry juice, diluted in a ratio of 1 to 10
— Weleda mouth water, diluted in a ratio of 1 to 50
— camomile tea

Wind a cotton cloth or a piece of gauze around your finger, moisten it with one of the above-mentioned solutions and get the baby to suck on this. Treat the breasts with this remedy after every feed as well (see also cracked nipples, p.59). If these remedies do not help, or if the baby is sick, has problems with drinking, diarrhea and/or a red bottom, consult the baby clinic about this problem in good time.

Also take a number of hygienic measures to prevent re-infection. Wash nappies, bibs, breast compresses and sheets at 90°C (194°F). Clean everything which comes into contact with the baby's mouth every day; don't forget your own hands.

The fungus which causes thrush can get into the baby's stools; it is a good idea to treat the bottom promptly with baby balm (Weleda), or zinc oil to prevent the baby's bottom from being affected. If the condition is accompanied by diarrhea, it is advisable to consult a doctor.

Spots on the face (milk spots or baby acne)
At first, spots on the face are very common. Usually, they disappear by themselves after a few weeks.

Teething
The baby's first teeth can be very painful. He will suddenly start to cry loudly, chew on everything, dribble a lot and may suffer from diarrhea and a red bottom. It is helpful to massage the gums or give the baby a teething ring and possibly some grains of Chamomilla radix D3.

Earache
If the child wakes up screaming in the night, grabbing hold of his ear, this could be a sign of an ear infection. The pain increases when the child is lying down. In many cases, the child will have been difficult and active before this at the end of the day. If you press on the bone just in front of the ear, this really hurts, which indicates that there is probably an ear infection.

The following measures are certainly worth trying: place an onion compress (see p.110) behind the painful red ear, and if possible hold it there for the night. Drip some physiological saline drops into the nostrils (see 'Blocked nose,' p.99); slightly raise the head end of the bed, for example, by placing a pillow under the mattress.

If the ear infection persists, you must call a doctor.

A snuffly baby
Children may suffer from a constant runny nose. This can be reduced by placing a slice of lemon under the feet, covered by a sock, by placing a sliced onion next to the bed or by dripping a physiological saline drops into the nostrils (see 'blocked nose,' p.99).

Coughs and colds
For these complaints, it is important that the child is warmly dressed, paying particular attention to the chest and back as regards warmth. In this case, woollen and silk underclothes are really essential (see p.27).

Drinking sage tea (made in the same way as ordinary tea) and rubbing the chest and back with thyme oil (Wala) can also be helpful.

Red bottom
When the child starts teething, his bottom may suddenly be bright red, and the skin can even be broken. This will disappear again when the teeth have come through completely.

In this case it is important to clean the bottom carefully with oil or water, to dry it thoroughly, possibly with a hair dryer and to apply baby balm (Weleda), mercurialis ointment (Weleda, Wala), zinc ointment or an ointment prescribed by the doctor. Different sorts of diapers (nappies) may also improve matters. If the condition is caused by thrush, you should consult the doctor.

Watery diapers (nappies)
If a child produces a large number of watery nappies every day, it has diarrhea and you should contact the doctor. This can be caused by gastroenteritis, teething or thrush. Babies in particular lose a lot of moisture and minerals when they have diarrhea, and this can result in dehydration.

When the nappies merely have thin stools, but not *watery* stools, it is possible to try some dietary measures first.

In principle, it is always possible to go on breastfeeding, even if the baby has diarrhea. If the baby is bottle fed, give it some extra liquid such as rice water and if the baby has cereals in the bottle or supplements, add rice flour or rice flakes. Puréed apple, banana, toast and rusks have a constipating effect, carrots are neutral.

Constipation
The child is constipated if the stools are hard and there are only sporadic stools in the diapers (nappies) at intervals of a few days, produced with a great deal of difficulty and sometimes pain. Babies which are only breastfed are never really constipated with hard stools, even though there may be no bowel movements for up to a week. It may happen with babies who are bottle fed. In this case, add some moisture and some extra oil (1 teaspoon of sunflower or olive oil to one bottle a day) or, if the child is ready for it, some orange juice or the water that prunes have been soaked in.

Cold feet
Small children often have cold feet and sometimes cold lower legs. This is not very desirable, as described earlier, p.24.

It helps to put on a pair of extra warm socks, rub the feet with copper ointment, or place a hot water bottle in the bed, removing it before putting the baby to bed. You can discuss this at the baby clinic.

Swimming for babies

In recent years, swimming has become very popular for babies. One of the reasons given for this is that children enjoy it so much. However, we question this obvious pleasure.

When a baby goes swimming it inevitably cools down a great deal. In addition, she is exposed to chlorinated water which has a damaging effect on her skin, so that there is an increased susceptibility to infection. The question also arises whether exposing a child to a large, often noisy, place is appropriate, as a young child obviously needs a sense of quiet security. Finally, there is plenty of time to enjoy swimming later on, when the child is a toddler.

Folic acid for a new pregnancy?

For over a decade, a campaign has been in place advising women who wanted to become pregnant to take folic acid tablets while trying to conceive and for the first three months of pregnancy. Taking folic acid was aimed at reducing the chances of having a child with spina bifida or other neural tube deficiencies.

The advice was to take a tablet of 0.4 mg of folic acid every day from four weeks before fertilization until twelve weeks after. In practice, this amounts to taking folic acid as soon you try to become pregnant. If you have an unplanned pregnancy, it is still possible to take these tablets for twelve weeks after fertilization. The tablets are available from chemists, pharmacists, health food shops, even supermarkets.

Women with an increased risk (see below) are also advised to take 0.4 mg, while women who have already had a child with spina bifida should take a higher dosage of folic acid, under the supervision of their doctor, midwife or gynaecologist. Multivitamin compounds are not advisable, unless prescribed by the doctor, because of the danger of overdosing on certain vitamins.

Not everyone will automatically want to follow this advice and start taking extra tablets for such a natural process as pregnancy. Nevertheless, it is impossible to ignore the option nowadays and when deciding whether or not to take the folic acid tablets, it may be helpful to be aware of a number of facts.

The chance of having a child with a spinal column defect, a defect in the development of the nervous system, is normally not very great at a very early stage of pregnancy. It occurs on average in 1 in 700 children.

The seriousness of this defect varies a great deal. In some of the children, the disorder is so serious that it is incompatible with life and the child only lives for a few days. Children who have spina bifida live with a handicap in the form of intestinal and bladder abnormalities and paralysis.

A number of factors play a role in the development of a defect in the spinal column and cord, though these are only partially understood. However, it is clear that hereditary factors play a role (the disorder is found in the family), and that the use of certain medicines for epilepsy or diabetes can result in an increased risk. These women have a so-called *increased* risk. In addition, the availability of certain foods also plays a role.

Research has shown that women who have already had a child with a defect in the spinal cord, and who take a fairly high dosage of folic acid during the first stage of their next pregnancy, have 70% less chance of having a child with the same disorder. Research on women taking folic acid without the risk factors, revealed a reduction in the chance of this disorder by 50%.

Folic acid is a vitamin in the vitamin B group, which is naturally found in many foods such as vegetables, fruit, cereals, pulses, dairy products and meat. It plays a role in the rapid division of cells in tissue. This obviously takes place in the developing child, and in adults, it plays a role in the mucus membranes of the intestines. It is not known exactly how the mechanism of folic acid works, but it is obvious that folic acid is essential.

The average European diet includes approximately 0.25 mg of folic acid per day. It is assumed that under normal circumstances this is sufficient. Under certain circumstances, for example, with the use of the contraceptive pill, the folic acid requirement is slightly increased. In view of the results of the above-mentioned research, the need for folic acid is probably also greater than 0.25 mg during pregnancy. The exact requirement is not known.

The advice assumes that 0.4 mg per day covers the extra need for folic acid, even in women with an increased risk. Women who have already had a child with a defect in the spinal cord are advised to take a much higher dosage, that is, 5 mg per day. It is assumed that these doses are not harmful. Certainly there are no known side effects. It is only when extremely high doses of folic acid were given in animal tests that there were harmful effects on the kidneys and nervous system.

Therefore, folic acid reduces the chance of a disorder but does not prevent it in all cases.

On the basis of the knowledge available at the moment, you will have to choose whether or not to take these folic acid tablets. For example, if you took the contraceptive pill before becoming pregnant, this could be an argument to take it. In cases of doubt, it is certainly a good idea to consult the doctor.

It is not an easy matter to achieve a dose of 0.4 mg through diet, in view of the quantities of vegetables and fruits which would have to be eaten. On the other hand, someone who did not want to take the tablets could take products rich in folic acid into account in their diet. These include broccoli, asparagus, sprouts, beetroot, strawberries, elderberries, buckthorn, berries, bananas, pears, oranges and wholewheat products. Like vitamin C, folic acid is sensitive to heat.

Appendix

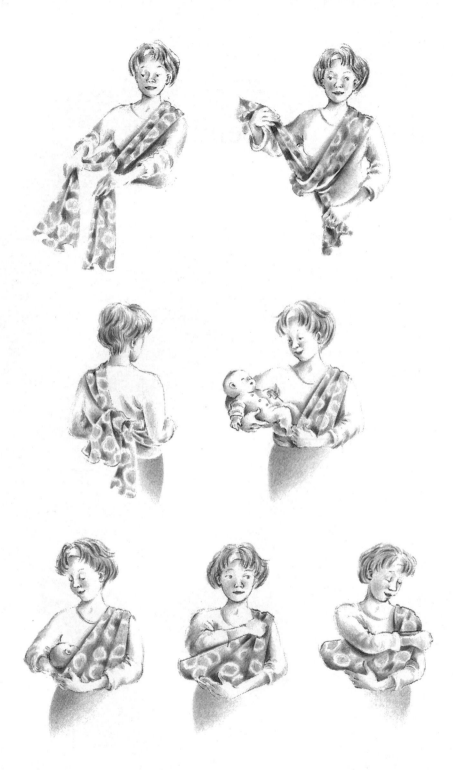

Procedures

Sling

1. Take a strong cotton cloth, 210 x 90 cm (80 x 36 in). Fold the cloth over one shoulder (if you are right handed over the left shoulder, if you are left handed over the right shoulder), and knot it with a strong knot on the opposite hip.
2. Move the knot onto your back until it is two thirds of the way up the back (in the hollow of your back).
3. Take the baby on the arm on the side where you have knotted the cloth.
4. Place the baby in the cloth with its stomach facing you. Place the baby's head on the edge of the cloth. Hold your arm under the baby until the baby is lying in the right place. Then move your arm from under the baby and support it with your other arm. Check that the knot on your back is still in the right place.
5. Raise the baby slightly with the carrying arm, and hold the side of the cloth that is next to the baby's neck.
6. Fold over the cloth by the neck back over your shoulder. This means that the baby's weight is distributed over the shoulder, so that carrying it does not put too much pressure on the neck. In addition, it means that the baby's head is in a slightly higher position.

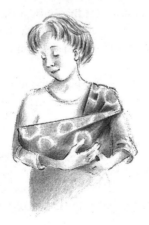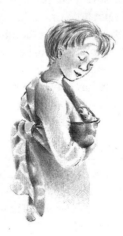

The first reaction of many parents is that the child is lying on the wrong side of the cloth, and can almost fall out of it. We have opted for this method because it is easier for the baby to get fresh air than with other methods. The danger that the baby will fall out is prevented by folding the cloth back over the shoulder. With this method it is a good idea to give the baby some support with the arm.

When you carry the baby, also look at your own position. Carrying a baby, even a light baby, with a hollow back will soon lead to problems. If the child moves down after being carried for a little, this can be corrected by pulling the cross over part of the cloth down slightly at the front, so that the head is automatically higher up.

Of course there are many other ways of tying a sling. There are baby slings on the market which give clear instructions.

Swaddling

Use a large, non-stretch cotton cloth
1. Fold one point in and place the baby on it, so that the fold in the piece of cloth falls just above the shoulders.
2. Move one arm down, slightly bent along the body, and fold the point of the cloth fairly tightly over the arm to the other side under the baby, so that the cloth is secured.
3. Now take the bottom point and place it diagonally across the baby up to the shoulder that has already been swaddled so that the cloth is also secured here. Make sure there is some room for the legs and hips.
4. Finally take hold of the last point and fold it firmly over the bent arm (so that the baby can find its thumb), or over the arm which has been bent down (see point 2) to the opposite side. Secure the cloth with one or more safety pins.
5. Experience has shown that very restless children who are swaddled with one arm pointing up will manage to undo the cloth. In that case it is better to swaddle both arms down.

Never place a swaddled child on his side, but always on his back. Make sure that the baby is not too warm, because a swaddled child will retain his own heat better. In principle, one layer of clothes under the swaddling clothes provide sufficient warmth. Then place the baby, firmly tucked in with a blanket, in a cot or bed.

Ways of folding diapers (nappies)

Three different ways of folding nappies are shown below.

Folding method 1

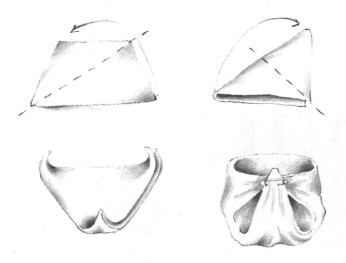

Folding method 2

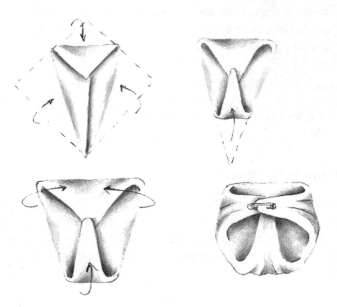

Folding method 3

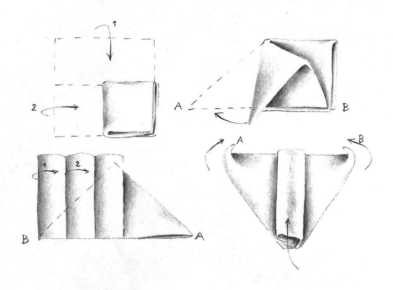

Camomile tea

Place one teaspoon of camomile flowers in a glass, and pour on boiling water. Leave the tea to brew for one minute. Then strain the tea and allow it to cool down. Give the tea with a spoon or in a bottle, or use it to clean the eyes or a blocked nose.

Fennel tea

Boil a few fennel seeds in water for about 5 minutes. The tea then has a pale yellow colour.

Onion compress for earache

Finely chop half an onion. Place the pieces on a cloth (for example a hand-kerchief), fold the cloth and stick it down with some elastoplast. Heat this package between a hot water bottle folded double or on a heater until it feels pleasantly warm. Place it on the child's ear and keep it in place with a bonnet.

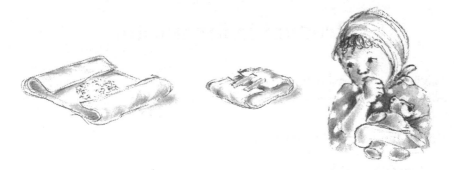

Camomile cloth for stomach cramps

Sprinkle some camomile oil on a cotton cloth the size of a postcard. Heat the cloth in a plastic bag between two hot water bottles. Also heat up a non-itchy woollen or flannel cloth.

Remove the warm compress from the plastic bag and place it on the stomach, wrapping the cloth around it and wrap the child up warmly. It can be left until the next time the baby is changed.

Walking round with a hot water bottle between yourself and the child, wrapped up in a warm cloth with a compress on her stomach, can also be very helpful.

Lemon wrap for a high fever

Squeeze half a lemon into a bowl of hot water with the palm of your hand. Soak the bandage in the lemon water. Ring out the bandage thoroughly and wrap around the child's feet and lower legs. The wrap must feel pleasantly warm to the child. Then put some woollen socks on the child.

Make sure that the child's feet are warm – if necessary, first place a warm hot water bottle at the bottom of the bed, but make sure that it is not over-heated.

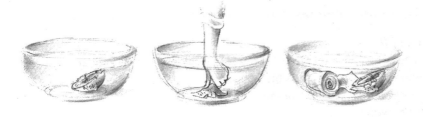

Product Information

The ingredients used in this book in the recipes for bottle-feeding and porridge are explained below in greater detail for each age.

Bottle-feeding 0–3 months

Full fat cow's milk
Try to use unhomogenized milk if possible, where the cream rises in the bottle so that there is a creamy layer at the top. Shake the bottle thoroughly or stir it before use.

Water
Do not use water from the boiler or hot water heater, but water from the cold water tap.

White almond paste and lactose
Both lactose and almond paste are available in most health shops.

Bottle-feeding 4–6 months

Types of flour
The types of flour that can be added to the bottle feed at this age are:
Rice flour
Organic baby flour from 4 months
Whole rice baby flour

Sweeteners
From five months it is possible to use a different sweetener instead of lactose; unprocessed sugar, baby malt, rice malt syrup or maple syrup.

Bottle-feeding and porridge 6–9 months

Types of flour
The choice depends on the baby's potential for digestion and pattern of excretion. At this age it is possible to use:
Organic baby flour from 6 months
3 cereals with spelt
wholewheat baby food

Sweetener
Unprocessed sugar, baby malt, rice or barley malt syrup or maple syrup

Oil
Cold-pressed sunflower oil

Porridge made of cereal flakes 6–9 months

Cereal flakes
Buy the flakes in small quantities at a time to make sure that they are fresh. Flakes which are suitable include rice, buckwheat, millet, oats and barley flakes. Oats and barley are the most difficult to digest.

Porridge 9–12 months

Types of flour
Wholewheat infant flour

Feeding Table

1-2 weeks: 6 to 8 times breast-feed (60 to 100 ml, 2-3.5 fl oz) per bottle-feed)
2-6 weeks: 6 to 7 times breast-feed (100 to 110 ml, 3.5-4 fl oz) per bottle-feed)
6-8 weeks: 5 to 6 times breast-feed (110 to 130 ml, 4-4.5 fl oz) per bottle-feed)
8-16 weeks: 4 to 5 times breast-feed (130 to 160 ml, 4.5-5.5 fl oz) per bottle-feed)

Weight gain during first year

From second month	150-250 g (6-9 oz) per week
From fourth month	130-200 g (5-7 oz) per week
From eight month	250-400 g (9-14 oz) per month

Weaning (for children with allergies begin after six months)

4 months (160-180 ml, 5.5-6.5 fl oz per feed)

early morning	breastfeed
late morning	fruit & breastfeed
afternoon	breastfeed
early evening	breastfeed
late evening	breastfeed

5 months (180-200 ml, 6.5-7 fl oz per feed)

early morning	breastfeed
late morning	vegetables & breastfeed
afternoon	fruit & breastfeed
early evening	breastfeed
late evening	breastfeed

5-6 months

early morning	breastfeed
late morning	vegetables, grains, 2 tsp oil & breastfeed
afternoon	fruit (& grains) & breastfeed
early evening	breastfeed
late evening	breastfeed

6 months

early morning	breastfeed
late morning	vegetables, grains and breastfeed
afternoon	fruit and breastfeed
early evening	porridge
evening	breastfeed

6 months

early morning	breastfeed
late morning	vegetables, grains and breastfeed
afternoon	fruit and breastfeed
early evening	porridge
evening	breastfeed
(late evening	breastfeed)

7 months

early morning	breastfeed (and porridge)
late morning	vegetables, grains, cheese/almond butter & yoghurt
afternoon	fruit, grains & breastfeed
early evening	porridge
evening	breastfeed

8 months

early morning	porridge and rusks
late morning	vegetables, grains, cheese/almond butter and dairy dessert
afternoon	fruit, grains and breastfeed
early evening	porridge
evening	breastfeed

from 9 months

early morning	porridge
late morning	some vegetables and dessert
afternoon	fruit and porridge or bread
late afternoon	porridge
early evening	breastfeed

from 10 to 12 months

early morning	porridge and/or bread
morning	snack
lunch	warm meal or bread and juice
afternoon	snack
evening	warm meal or porridge

We recommend breastfeeding. However, in the above scheme at each place where breastfeed is recommended, bottle can be given instead.

Bibliography

Health and sickness

Bentheim, T van, *Home Nursing for Carers,* Floris Books, Edinburgh 2006.

Bie, Guus van der and Huber, Machteld, *Foundations of Anthroposophical Medicine,* Floris Books, Edinburgh 2003.

Bott, Victor, *Anthroposophical Medicine,* Anthroposophic Press, New York.

Bühler, Walter, *Living with your Body: the Body as an Instrument of the Soul,* Rudolf Steiner Press, London.

Evans, Michael and Rodger, Iain, *Healing for Body, Soul: An Introduction to Anthroposophical Medicine,* Floris Books, Edinburgh 2000. IN USA published as *Complete Healing,* Steinerbooks, New York 2007.

Glöcker, Michaela and Goebel, Wolfgang, *A Guide to Child Health,* Floris Books, Edinburgh, 2007.

Holtzapfel, Walter, *Children's Destinies: the Three Directions of Human Development,* Mercury Press, New York.

—, *Our Children's Illnesses,* Mercury Press, New York.

Husemann, Armin, *The Harmony of the Human Body,* Floris Books, Edinburgh 2002.

Leroi, Rita, *Illness and Healing,* Temple Lodge Press, London.

Leviton, Richard, *Anthroposophic Medicine Today,* Anthroposophic Press, New York.

Mees, L.F.S. *Blessed by Illness,* Anthroposophic Press, New York.

Steiner, Rudolf, *Introducing Anthroposophical Medicine,* Anthroposophical Press, New York.

Steiner, Rudolf, and Ita Wegman, *The Fundamentals of Therapy,* Rudolf Steiner Press, London.

Studer, Hans-Peter and Douch, Geoffrey, *Vaccination, A Guide for Making Personal Choices,* Floris Books, Edinburgh 2004.

Twentyman, Ralph, *The Science and Art of Healing,* Floris Books, Edinburgh 1992.

Wolff, Otto, *Anthroposophically Orientated Medicine and its Remedies,* Mercury Press, New York.

—, *Home Remedies,* Floris Books, Edinburgh 2000.

Babies and toddlers

Blom, Ria, *Crying and Restlessness in Babies,* Floris Books, Edinburgh 2005.

Gibson, Margaret, *Becoming a Mother,* Hale & Iremonger, Sydney.

Glas, Norbert, *Conception, Birth and Early Childhood,* Anthroposophic Press, New York.

Gotsch, Gwen and Judy Torgus, *The Womanly Art of Breastfeeding,* La Lèche League International, Illionois 1997.

König, Karl, *The First Three Years of the Child,* Floris Books, Edinburgh 1998.

Mitchell, Ingrid, *Breastfeeding Together,* Seabury Press, New York 1978.

Linden, Wilhelm zur, *A Child is Born,* Rudolf Steiner Press, London.

Parenting & general education

Anschütz, Marieke, *Children and their Temperaments,* Floris Books, Edinburgh 1995.

Being a Parent, Parent Network, Hawthorn Press, Stroud.

Britz-Crecelius, Heidi, *Children at Play,* Inner Traditions, Vermont.

Dunn, Judy, and Robert Plomin. *Separate Lives: Why Siblings Are So Different,* Basic Books, 1990.

Harwood, A.C. *The Way of a Child,* Sophia Books, Forest Row.

Kane, Franklin G. *Parents as People: the Family as a Creative Process,* Aurora, Edmonton.

Kiel-Hinrichsen, Monika, *Why Children don't Listen,* Floris Books, Edinburgh 2006.

König, Karl, *Brothers and Sisters: the Order of Birth in the Family,* Floris Books, Edinburgh.

Maslow, Abraham H. *Motivation and Personality,* Harper & Row, New York, 1987.

Needleman, H. L., and P. J. Landrigan, *Raising Children Toxic Free,* Farrar, Straus & Giroux, New York 1994.

Pearce, Joseph Chilton, *The Magical Child,* Bantam, New York.

Salter, Joan, *The Incarnating Child,* Hawthorn Press, Stroud.

Useful Organizations

Immunization

Government recommended schedules

UK: www.immunisation.nhs.uk
Ireland: www.immunisation.ie
USA: http://mchb.hrsa.gov/mchirc/chusa
Canada: www.phac-aspc.gc.ca
Australia: www.mydr.com.au
New Zealand: www.immune.org.nz
South Africa: www.capegateway.gov.za

Anthroposophical medicine

Physicians' Association for Anthroposophic Medicine (PAAM)
1923 Geddes Ave, Ann Arbor MI48104
Tel: 734-930-9462 Fax: 734-662-1727
Email: paam@anthroposophy.org
www.paam.net

The Anthroposophical Medical Association
53 Cainscross Road, Stroud GL5 4EX
Tel: 01453-762 151
Email: medical.section@yahoo.co.uk

Park Attwood Clinic
Trimpley, Bewdley, Worcs. DY12 1RE
Tel: 01299-861 444 Fax: 01299-861 375
www.parkattwood.org

Weleda
Heanor Road, Ilkeston DE7 8DR **UK**
Tel: 0115-944 8222

Fax: 0115-944 8210
Email: Weleda.direct@weleda.co.uk
www.weleda.co.uk

PO Box 675, Palisades NY 10964 **US**
Tel: 800-241-1030
Fax: 800-280-4899
Email: info@weleda.com
http://usa.weleda.com

302 Te Mata Road, Havelock North **NZ**
Tel. 0800-802 174
Fax: 0800-804 989
Email: weleda@weleda.co.nz
www.weleda.co.nz

Australia Tel: 03-9723 7278
Email: weleda@weleda.com.au

Pharma Natura **(South Africa)**
PO Box 494, Bergvlei 2012
Tel: 011-445 6000 Fax: 011-445 6089
Email: healthcare@pharma.co.za
www.pharma.co.za

International
Anthroposophical Society Medical Section, Goetheanum, 4143 Dornach, Switzerland
Tel: +41-61-706 4290
Fax: +41-61-706 4291
Email: am@medsektion-goetheanum.ch
www.medsektion-goetheanum.org

Childbirth, breastfeeding

La Leche League (Great Britain)
PO Box 29, West Bridgford, Nottingham, NG2 7NP
Tel. 0845-456-1855
www.laleche.org.uk

La Leche League International
PO Box 4079, Schaumburg IL, 60168–4079
Tel. 847-519-7730
Fax: 847-969-0460
www.llli.org

National Childbirth Trust
Oldham Terrace, London W3 6NH
Enq: 0870-444 8707
Fax: 0870-770 3237
Breastfeeding Line: 0870-444 8708
www.nct.org.uk

Index

Michaela Glöckler & Wolfgang Goebel

A Guide to Child Health

Third Edition

Now in its third edition, this revised and updated guide to children's physical, psychological and spiritual development combines medical advice with issues of upbringing and education.

Throughout, the book is extremely practical, covering all childhood illnesses, ailments and conditions, and home nursing. The authors also outline the connection between education and healing, with all that this implies for the upbringing and good health of children. Medical, educational and religious questions often overlap, and in the search for the meaning of illness it is necessary to study the child as a whole — as body, soul and spirit.

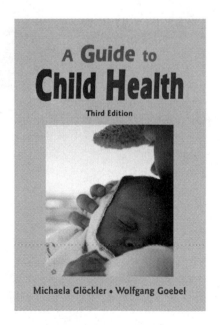

'A vital book for parents who seek a deeper understanding of their child's health. 'The Green Parent Favourite' award.'
—*The Green Parent*

'Full of the kind of wise tips that used to get passed down from mother to daughter but are sadly missing in this day and age. An invaluable reference source. Highly recommended.'
— *Juno: A natural approach to family life*

www.florisbooks.co.uk